Comfort Theory and Practice

A Vision for Holistic Health Care and Research

Dear Anne, Thanks for listening & thinking about Comfort Theory. May you experience comfort in your own life as well.

Best wishes,
Kathy Kolcaba
5/22/07

Katharine Kolcaba, PhD, RN, C, is an Associate Professor at The University of Akron College of Nursing, where she enjoys teaching Comfort Care at different student levels. In addition to teaching theory, she also specializes in gerontology, research, and community health. She is the coordinator of her local Parish Nurse program (see chapter 9), and provided leadership in developing the college's Nursing Care of Older Adults course, which won first place in a national competition sponsored by the Association of American Colleges of Nursing and the Hartford Foundation for Gerontological Excellence. Kolcaba has published extensively on the patient outcome of holistic comfort (see References), including an award-winning Web site called The Comfort Line.

Comfort Theory and Practice

A Vision for Holistic Health Care and Research

Katharine Kolcaba, PhD, RN, C

 Springer Publishing Company

Springer Publishing Company, Inc.
536 Broadway
New York, NY 10012-3955

Acquisitions Editor: Ruth Chasek
Production Editor: J. Hurkin-Torres
Cover Design by Joanne Honigman
Cover Art by David Jansen
Chapter Illustrations by Karen Crabtree, except chapter 8 by David Jansen.

Library of Congress Cataloging-in-Publication Data

Kolcaba, Katharine.
    Comfort theory and practice : a vision for holistic health care and research / Katharine Kolcaba.
        p. cm.
    Includes bibliographical references and index.
    ISBN 0-8261-1663-7
    1. Holistic medicine.   2. Alternative medicine.   I. Title.
    R733 .K584 2003
    610—dc21
                                                            2002075860
                                                            CIP

Printed in Canada by Tri-Graphics Printing (Ottawa) Limited.

On September 11th, 2001, Lynn Slepski, MSN, RN, was ready. Her job as Commander, U.S. Public Health Service, was to order the mobilization of emergency supplies along with medical and nursing personnel to any major disaster site in the United States. When the second plane hit the South Tower of the World Trade Center in New York City, the loaded Navy hospital ship was deployed immediately. The name of the ship was . . . *Comfort.*

Adapted from Kennedy, M. (2002). Nurses making a difference: Our worst disaster's first nurse. *American Journal of Nursing, 102*(2), 102–103.

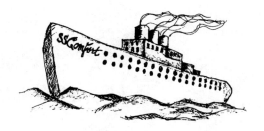

Contents

List of Figures

List of Tables and Case Studies

TABLES

CASE STUDIES

Foreword

D r. Katharine Kolcaba has been working on the outcome of patient comfort since 1987 when she started her PhD studies at Case Western Reserve University. Her record of publications chronicle the process of concept development for her Comfort Theory. Dr. Kolcaba begins this publication, *Comfort Theory and Practice: A Vision for Holistic Health Care and Research,* by defining comfort from the patients' perspective, then discussing the measurement system used to validate this concept, its importance and placement within the context of a theory for health care, and the evolution of the theory for the 21st century. The book provides a blueprint for application of Comfort Theory in practice, education, research, and quality improvement.

Providing comfort to the patient is an integral part of nursing. Comfort encompasses the integration of concern for the spiritual, emotional, and physical aspects of patient care. According to Dr. Kolcaba, patient comfort is a very complex, rich, valued, and useful concept for health care. The strengthening property of comfort is especially important for patients who are trying to return to former functional levels, who are going through strenuous therapies or rehabilitation programs, or who want to die in a dignified way. As suggested by Dr. Kolcaba in the Theory of Comfort, patients who are comfortable do better and they heal more quickly, saving precious health care dollars.

Enhanced comfort, as an immediate desirable outcome of nursing care, is theoretically correlated with desirable health seeking behaviors. Health seeking behaviors of patients, in turn, are positively related to Institutional Integrity (values, financial stability, and wholeness of health care organizations). As health care organizations strive to maintain a high level of care with shrinking human and financial resources, the Comfort Care approach provides a cost-effective model for these organizations. The framework of this model offers nurses and other health care team members a guideline for holistic assessment and a design for intervention, evaluation, and for patient care planning.

Dr. Kolcaba also advocates for the creation of work environments that provide an atmosphere of comfort for nurses, who will then have the resources to enhance patient comfort (this is covered in chapter 9). Comfort for nurses entails autonomy, staffing in concert with best practice models, administrative support, continuing education, and compassionate mentoring, to name a few components.

I am honored and delighted to recommend this text for all nurses and health care providers who care for and care about patients.

MAY WYKLE, RN, PhD, FAAN
Dean, The Frances Payne Bolton School of Nursing
Case Western Reserve University
Cleveland, Ohio

Preface

This book is a compilation of work about the outcome of patient comfort. It presents, in one easy-to-use text, the various segments of work about comfort arranged topically and in the chronological order in which they occurred. I have tried to make the book personal, user-friendly, and confidence-building for nurses and other health care team members who think that a comfort-oriented, theory-based practice is a good idea for patients, practitioners, and health care organizations.

In addition to my own work, a lengthy reference list at the end of the book is evidence of many other authors from nursing and related disciplines who have contributed to my building of the Comfort Theory. No theory occurs in a vacuum, and the Theory of Comfort especially was created out of a renewed collective consciousness about the importance of comfort in health care. While I did not realize it at the time I was developing the theory, in retrospect I see clearly that there was a rich context in health care and graduate education in the United States providing me with frequent helpmates and "lightbulbs" regarding insights about patient comfort. I tried to recreate this context here, to show that anyone can tune in and bring ideas together.

Writing this book has given me a chance to reexamine the consistency of Comfort Theory, and its implications and applications. During this examination, I have acquired new insights and ideas about the possibilities of comfort. I have also enjoyed the interactive thinking that occurs during composition—a sort of writer's system of checks and balances. So this has been a rewarding time of integration, discussion, and refinement in which new ideas emerged in light of changes in health care and global realities. After all these years with Comfort Theory, I didn't think it would still grow. This speaks to the dynamics of the concept, our language, the discipline of nursing and health care in general, and my desire to capture the nuances of comfort.

My editor wanted this book to be oriented toward practicing nurses and I agreed. Nurses are the main consumers of the theory and if they can't use it or understand it, Comfort Theory will fade away. So, above all, this book is for nurses. I also have taken my editor's request a few steps further as work on the book and life events unfolded. The first step beyond what was requested occurred because of some outside invitations received during the writing of the book. When I thought about what I would present to these national groups, I came to realize that Comfort Care (my title for Comfort Theory when it is *applied*) is not limited to nursing. True, it began in nursing and I am proud of its traditional roots, as you will see in the book. But it can be an interdisciplinary model for health care, and I sincerely hope this will happen in the future. Comfort Care can unify health care practice because it is oriented to the one thing those disciplines have in common: patients. Any practitioner who works with patients or groups in need of health care, whether it is prevention, safety, management of chronic illnesses, treatment of acute episodes, or at the beginning or end of life, can use the framework of Comfort Care. Because I think that interdisciplinary health care *is* the future, I think it would be easier if we were all on the same page.

The second step beyond what was requested occurred after I attended a presentation about staffing issues in hospitals. The presenter was Peter Buerhaus, the nurse-statistician who has been instrumental in doing nursing outcomes research. He has been able to demonstrate that nurses make valuable contributions to patient outcomes. He and the articles he has written have convinced me that practicing nurses will be participating in Quality Improvement (QI) *of their own practices.* Nurse educators will be teaching these techniques in academic settings and in-service programs. By definition, QI requires documentation and measurement of positive and negative patient outcomes related to nursing and/or interdisciplinary care. The idea, of course, is to *decrease* the negative and *increase* the positive patient outcomes on your unit!

Certainly, comfort is a positive patient outcome and I hope all nurses and other team members will claim it as one they want to enhance and document. Nurses can and should use the standardized, computerized data sets available to nursing for their QI demonstrations (more about these data sets in chapter 9); but the important point here is that nursing and interdisciplinary care will no longer be disengaged from research. Rather, a part of our everyday practice will be to measure outcomes, although it may be called something else so as not to sound too overwhelming. Therefore, this book integrates practice and research throughout and, I hope, serves as a guide for blending health care with outcomes research.

The third step beyond what was requested by my editor occurred as a result of the terrorist attacks of September 11, 2001. The attacks occurred as I was gearing up for my final chapter, wondering how it would turn out. Thus, in chapter 10 I reflect on America's new heroes, on how we can comfort each other in the face of peril, and on the human need for comfort. Also in this chapter are my hopes for peace, cooperation, understanding, tolerance, and (yes) comfort for our global neighbors. The book ends with a "mythic vision" for comfort around the world—it is a vision that I hope readers will consider keeping in their heads and working toward.

For now, thank you for being a reader. May you feel inclined to become a member of our Comfort Team in any of a variety of ways. In your practice, as you teach, as you live, and as you wrestle with research or ethical problems, may comfort be in your future.

Kathy Kolcaba

Acknowledgments

The writing of this book was accomplished only through much love and support. First, this book is a tribute to you, my students and fellow colleagues, my contacts from the Internet, and all users of Comfort Theory. Because of your feedback and requests, I was motivated to put everything I currently understand or have done regarding patient comfort into one convenient text. Now you can get everything you need for your assignments, clinical initiatives, or research, from this book. No searching for articles and no copying costs (I remember what that's like!). Here's hoping, therefore, that this book will be a handy reference for all of you who might be interested in using the Comfort Theory in one way or another, either now or in the future.

Secondly, I was supported in this endeavor by many. My editor at Springer Publishing, Ruth Chasek, was kind, prompt, skillful, and decisive. The Dean of the College of Nursing at the University of Akron, Dr. Cynthia Capers, granted me a sabbatical for the purpose of writing this book. In this and many other ways, she demonstrated that she believed in what I was doing with comfort. Our college's technical support person, John Gurnak, kept me going when some nasty viruses had other ideas. My son-in-law, Rick VanDerveer, *made* me back up my files—Wow! That was timely, book-saving support! My son-in-law, Dave Jansen, also contributed by sensitively rendering the cover art. My dear friend and research partner, Dr. Therese Dowd, argued with and cajoled me about comfort, helped me apply it with patients and students, and edited the rough drafts of these chapters thoughtfully and carefully. And to Karen Crabtree, my illustrator, friend, and nurse who added her talents to the chapters: a big hug for understanding what I wanted to convey in pictures.

During graduate education, my professors at Case Western Reserve University presented me with the right challenges at the right time and extra support when needed. Dr. May Wykle, in particular, was always a paragon of comfort for me, a mentor in every sense; she was my lion who defended my holistic ideas when holism wasn't very popular. My first statistics professor, Dr. Richard Steiner, continues to demonstrate the art of statistical analysis to me and he really appreciates the complexities of measuring patient comfort. The Alumni Association at the Frances Payne Bolton School of Nursing and Sigma Theta Tau (Alpha Mu and Delta Omega chapters) supported me with funding at crucial periods in my career. To all of these people and organizations, I will be forever grateful.

My family is my respite and my grounding and I thank them from the bottom of my heart for always being there for me. My mom first introduced me to comfort with her unconditional love and assurance of possibilities for my future that had no limits based on gender or age or income. She is a model of perseverance. My philosopher-husband, Raymond, helped me write my first article when I was newly graduated from my MSN program (15 years ago) and he continues to be enthusiastic about patient comfort and an invaluable problem solver. For this project he contributed significantly to chapters 6 and 8. He truly understands and believes in comfort! My daughters, Christine, Jill, and Liz, and my seven grandchildren have been my cheerleaders and my reminders to live in the present moment. Their health and vitality enable and inspire me.

Lastly, this book is dedicated to the memory of my brother, John Arnold, III, and my father, John Arnold, Jr. Both died too young and are missed deeply these many years later—but they smile at me, encourage me in my dreams, and I believe that I will see them again.

Thank you, one and all.

CHAPTER 1

The Seeds of Inquiry

Comfort may be a blanket or breeze,
some ointment here to soothe my knees;
A listening ear to hear my woes,
a pair of footies to warm my toes;
A PRN medication to ease my pain,
someone to reassure me once again;
A call from my doctor, or even a friend,
a rabbi or priest as my life nears the end.
Comfort is whatever I perceive it to be,
a necessary thing defined only by me.
—S. D. Lawrence (student nurse)
(Kolcaba, 1995b, p. 289)

Patient comfort and comfort care are complicated, individual, and holistic concepts. I began my exploration of these topics about 15 years ago, after "discovering" the concepts through my nursing practice. After the discovery and explication phases, many years were devoted to analyzing, defining, operationalizing, theorizing, and testing the extent of patient comfort under different circumstances. This chapter begins with a brief autobiography describing where I was when this endeavor began and why I undertook it. I then discuss the details of where the exploration took me, from explaining "comfort" in common language, to defining comfort as an outcome of nursing, to applying comfort in interdisciplinary health care. The details culminate with the taxonomic structure of comfort, a diagram of the content domain, and a technical definition for this rich and multidimensional concept. The taxonomic structure laid the foundation for all the subsequent work, as will become evident in later chapters. Lastly, in this and every chapter, I muse about the comfort quote at the beginning of each chapter.

A BRIEF AUTOBIOGRAPHY

I was born in Cleveland, Ohio and spent most of my life in this city. In 1965, I received a diploma in nursing from St. Luke's Hospital School of Nursing in Cleveland. I practiced full and part time for many years in medical surgical nursing, long-term care, and home care while raising my three daughters. In the mid 1980s, my daughters were becoming self sufficient and I yearned for a promotion—which required an academic degree. After extensive decision making and fulfilling of pre-requisites, I entered the Frances Payne Bolton School of Nursing, Case Western Reserve University (CWRU). In 1987, I graduated in the first RN to MSN class, with a specialty in gerontology. While going to school, I job-shared a head nurse position on a dementia unit. In the context of that unit and my MSN coursework, I began theorizing about the outcome of comfort.

Following graduation, I joined the faculty at The University of Akron (UA) College of Nursing. Because it was a job requirement, I began the pursuit of my doctorate in nursing at CWRU on a part-time basis while continuing to teach full time. Over the next 10 years, I utilized coursework from my doctoral program and feedback from students at CWRU and UA to develop and explicate the Theory of Comfort. I graduated with a PhD in Nursing in 1997.

More Than an Assignment

As so often happens in life, a seminal event occurred early in my academic career. Perhaps because it was one of my first courses, I did not recognize the importance of that class at the time; but my 15-year (so far) exploration of the concept of comfort for nursing actually began with an assignment from Dr. Rosemary Ellis, in a course called Introduction to Nursing Theory. She asked us to diagram our nursing practice, a deceptively easy-sounding task. We were to include concepts specific to our setting that were in the literature. These concepts were to be put into a succinct diagram with directional arrows and positive and negative signs denoting relationships between those concepts. This assignment challenged us to think about our nursing practice, what we hoped patients in a specific setting would accomplish, and how we helped to bring about those goals. Putting all of this information into a succinct diagram was an exercise in precise thinking, and in tribute to Dr. Ellis, a brilliant undertaking to ask of us. (I have since used this assignment in my own teaching of MSN students and have had wonderful, creative, thought-provoking student posters as a result.) So began the intense introspection about my nursing style and values, as they applied to my current setting.

PRACTICE SETTING FOR THE FIRST COMFORT DIAGRAM

At the time, in the late 1980s, I held the position of head nurse on an Alzheimer's unit. There were many things I loved about dementia care, but one interesting aspect that shaped my response to Ellis's assignment was that my 15 residents were nonverbal in the customary sense. They did talk, but usually in the form of "word salads" or, in the later stages of dementia, familiar sounds put together in non-English ways. Moreover, theirs was a fragile existence because any "minor" physical or emotional change could disrupt their equilibrium resulting in displays of excess disabilities (EDs). EDs were previously defined in dementia care as reversible symptoms that are undesirable and temporary extensions of a specific primary disability (Schwab, Rader, & Doan, 1985). Examples of excess disabilities are agitation, fighting with others, refusal to cooperate, temper tantrums, or tearing apart the environment. Primary disabilities can result from the compromise of any organ system, an injury, an infection, an emotional trauma, dehydration, or constipation. When one of our residents displayed an ED, the entire unit was soon disrupted, as one resident's agitation caused the others to be agitated as well. It was *important*, therefore, to prevent or treat excess disabilities as efficiently as possible.

Our problem, of course, was that when our residents had a physical or mental disability, they couldn't tell us what was wrong. We had to be detectives, surmising the problem from the residents' body language, their long-term health and emotional history, what they were doing or had done that day, who had visited, and any risk factors to which they were prone. For example, a mild urinary tract infection could result in agitation but no other symptoms. (We ran a lot of "chemsticks" on that unit!) At any rate, in the absence of sophisticated verbal communication, we became very sensitive to the residents' needs and backgrounds.

The First Article: The Concept of Comfort in an Environmental Framework

I was familiar with the current terms used to describe the practice of dementia care. In addition to EDs, *facilitative environment* and *optimum function* were discussed frequently. These three terms were the foundation of my diagram and I drew relationships between them for the assignment. Facilitative environment is the therapeutic milieu which is adapted to address the needs of frail patients (Wolanin & Phillips, 1981).

In the diagram, I subdivided the manifestations of EDs into physical and psychological, because in practice our detective work began by examining these two different but interrelated causes. Then I pondered about what we were doing on our unit to prevent EDs. These nursing actions that were taken to prevent or treat EDs were called interventions or comfort measures.

Optimum function had been conceptualized as the ability to engage in special activities on the unit (Wolanin & Phillips, 1981), such as setting the table, getting bathed and dressed, preparing a salad, or sitting through a program. These activities did not happen more than twice a day because the residents couldn't tolerate much more than that. What were the residents doing in the mean time? In what state of normalcy did I, the head nurse, want them to be before and after tasks of optimal function were performed? What behaviors did the staff and I want them to exhibit that would indicate an *absence* of EDs? What could I call this state that seemed so important to my nursing practice and which my residents, because of their dementia, could not articulate?

After long discussions and musings with my philosopher-husband, Dr. Ray Kolcaba, the word "comfort" came to me. This concept, as I understood its ordinary meaning, described very well the desirable state we wanted for our residents most of the time. The term itself represented a relaxed, healthy, peaceful, and *individualized* condition for each resident. When my residents were in a state of comfort (comfortable) they socialized informally with others, wandered casually, sat easily, napped, cooperated with staff, laughed, or hummed, and generally displayed ease and contentment within their surroundings.

Moreover, this state of comfort seemed to be a necessary condition for those special tasks that required optimum function. Being comfortable before doing something difficult seemed to give our residents the where-withal to pull themselves together, to call upon old patterns of social grace and behaviors so that they could fit in with other residents during special programs. I became excited about the ability of the concept of comfort to capture this elusive and important state for my residents and I introduced the term to the original diagram. This word seemed to convey the desired state for patients to be in when they were not engaging in special activities and before they could engage in these activities.

Composing this framework marked the first steps towards a theory of comfort and my emerging thoughts about the complexities of the concept (Figure 1.1). By the time this assignment was finished, Dr. Ellis was quite ill and unable to continue teaching. She took the time, however, to refer me to Dr. Mary Adams for help in converting my framework to a paper. When I showed Dr. Adams the framework, she responded immediately, "Comfort? You're interested in comfort? That

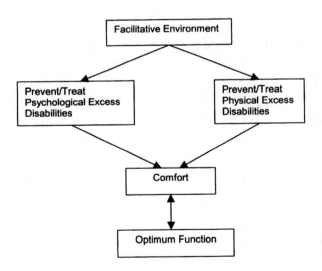

FIGURE 1.1   A framework of care for gerontological nursing.

Kolcaba, K. (1992a). The concept of comfort in an environmental framework. *Journal of Gerontological Nursing, 18*(6), 33–38. (Reprinted by permission of Slack Corporation.)

is such a beautiful nursing concept—you should really pursue your work with comfort." I was surprised and happy, but certainly very naïve about what "working with comfort" would entail. Because it was not required at the time, I had not defined comfort and I truly did not know the ramifications of using this concept in my diagram. Furthermore, I was far from being committed to any further work with comfort.

Before I graduated from my MSN program, I submitted an abstract describing my framework for dementia care to a gerontological conference in Toronto. (My CWRU professors encouraged us to do this sort of thing.) When the abstract was accepted, I really began to sweat. It would be my first nursing conference, I was a new MSN graduate, and I didn't know what to expect—except that I would be the new kid on the block, with a framework that might or might not be interesting to experienced nurses.

The First Conference: University of Toronto Gerontological Conference

Like most nursing conferences, the one in Toronto produced feedback that was thoughtful and thought provoking. One observation from the audience was that the framework was applicable to many nursing settings and did not have to be limited in its scope to dementia care. The question from the audience, however, that shaped the rest of my career was, "Have you done a concept analysis of comfort?" At the time I barely knew what a concept analysis was, let alone realized the importance of doing it for the complex concept of comfort. I gulped, and answered, "No, but that is my next step." ("Where did that come from?" I wondered, as I hadn't decided to go back to school.)

The conference went well because the experienced nurses made me feel welcome. I left the conference uneasily, though, feeling committed to fulfilling the "promise" I had made to the anonymous person in the audience—to actually do a concept analysis of comfort, which I didn't know how to do. It took 2 years to write and publish the framework (Kolcaba, 1992a), but the resultant article gave me encouragement to keep going with my work with comfort.

CONCEPT ANALYSIS

When I returned from Toronto, I began to seriously think about proceeding with a concept analysis of comfort. Because I had not yet enrolled in a PhD program, however, I needed help. Fortunately, my husband specialized in epistemology, the theory of knowledge, and he knew how to do a concept analysis. As my first assignment, he told me to find ways in which comfort was used in nursing and in all other disciplines that we would expect to use it. Thus began an extensive review of the literature about comfort from the disciplines of nursing, medicine, psychology, theology, psychiatry, and ergonomics. I also looked at contemporary and archaic uses of comfort in English, including its use by Shakespeare, who loved the term in all its forms. Webster's (1979) dictionary alone revealed six different definitions of comfort.

In nursing, a rich historical record of the use of comfort was found in Nightingale's *Notes on Nursing* (1859), old textbooks, new textbooks, and in the writing of nurse theorists. Nursing diagnoses at that time focused on "altered comfort" and named three specific detractors from comfort: pain, nausea/vomiting, and itching (Carpenito, 1987). This trend of discussing comfort in terms of its detractors was exemplified in a 1988 conference entitled *Key Aspects of Comfort: Management of Pain, Fatigue, and Nausea,* the proceedings of which were published in a book of the same title (Funk, Tornquist, Champagne, Copp, & Wiese, 1989). In contemporary nursing textbooks, the importance of patient comfort was noted, but usually then discussed as pain management.

During the discovery phase of our concept analysis, an important component of comfort emerged from three sources, which was to be central to its importance for nursing: its strengthening component. The first source of this component was in its word origin, the Latin word "confortare," meaning to strengthen greatly. The second source was from Paterson (Paterson & Zderad, 1976/1988) who stated that comfort freed patients to be all that they could be at the time, a belief that conformed to the archaic origin of the term. The third source to speak to the strengthening component of comfort was disciplinary. Ergonomics and psychology were interested in enhancing productivity, efficiency, or performance when specific tasks were required. The way to increase performance was to increase the comfort of the worker or athlete through manipulating the environment, the furniture, the psychological messages, et cetera. Enhanced comfort, therefore, strengthened or inspired the worker or athlete to "do better" (Kendall, Hrycaido, & Martino, 1990; Lee, 1990; McClelland, 1988; Suin, 1972). Discovering that comfort, in its origins and in its usage in other disciplines, entailed a strengthening component was exciting, because it provided a later rationale for nurses and other team members to enhance patients' comfort, beyond the altruistic reasons advocated by nursing theorists.

The Second Article: The Concept Analysis

Adding to the complexity of the concept analysis was the fact that comfort could be a verb, noun, gerund (comforting), adjective (comfortable), process or product (outcome), and in past, present, or future tense. The next 2 years were spent making sense of all these usages and parts of speech, then organizing the findings.

In the process of producing an article for nursing, the different writing and working styles of my husband and myself emerged. I tend to work quickly, impatiently, and imperfectly on the computer. I don't like details, and want to get things "off my desk." I think in overviews and whole pictures, am creative, and can usually find a way to compromise, get outside a box and move on. My husband takes just the opposite approach. Ray takes months to dwell on subject matter, does most of the work in his head, and only after much philosophizing does he discuss his conclusions or put them down on paper. I would find a lot of citations where comfort was used, show them to my husband, and wait for him to sort mentally through their meanings and applications before discussing them with me. Putting conclusions onto paper is laborious and time consuming for him. He strives for perfection with every draft—while I count on editors to help reach that goal.

Thus, our first (and only) coauthored article about comfort took about 2 years to complete, patience I didn't know I had, and a dedication to comfort that my husband needed to cultivate. The resulting article was complicated, intense, and hard to publish because much of the language was laced with difficult philosophical terms and phrases that my husband used in his own discipline and about which he would not compromise. We submitted and resubmitted the article to several American journals, only to have reviews such as, "This gives me a headache." When we submitted the manuscript to publishers in Great Britain, however, it found ready acceptance in the *Journal of Advanced Nursing*. Their only request was to make the ending more exciting, something I eagerly did. Comfort was off and running in nursing, and Ray, tired and saturated with comfort, said "No more." To this day, I find that article (Kolcaba & Kolcaba, 1991) complex and difficult to read, but thorough and accurate. Moreover, it has stood the test of time.

After we had completed our concept analysis (but before we found a publishing home), we sent an abstract to Sigma Theta Tau International for presentation in Indiana. In the abstract, I proposed to define the concept of comfort for nursing, which was a simplified but natural extension of the concept analysis. When the abstract was accepted, I reworked the analysis to arrive at three types of comfort that were relevant and current in nursing.

THREE TYPES OF COMFORT

The three technical senses of comfort that we presented at Sigma Theta Tau (STT) were *relief, ease,* and *renewal;* the term renewal was later changed to transcendence. *Relief* was defined then as the experience of a patient who has had a specific comfort need met. *Ease* was defined as a state of calm or contentment. Renewal (*transcendence*) was defined as the state in which one rises above problems or pain. The article that presented these three types of comfort, plus subsequent work on holism, took another 2 years to write and publish (Kolcaba, 1991).

The Second Conference: Sigma Theta Tau

What would our audience at STT think of these types of comfort? Would they disagree with the findings or come up with something different? This would be the first time our analysis would be under public and disciplinary scrutiny and I was uneasy about this "test." Therefore, I asked Ray to accompany me for the presentation, a legitimate request as he was second author on the abstract.

I presented our paper. The audience reaction was strong, and frankly, hostile. "Why are you making comfort so complicated? We all know what it means!" This was exactly what I was afraid of, as I had no résumé of articles and very few academic credentials to back me up. Ray was able to address those complaints comfortably, however, with the confidence of being a philosopher and educator for 20 years; "If your discipline is going to progress as a science, you must define your central terms precisely so you can understand each other and develop ways to conduct research about them." (Dr. Ellis had said the same thing 5 years previous to this but I had not recalled her words during the presentation.) Ray continued, "All disciplines must define their concepts. We have demonstrated that 'comfort' is used in many ways and has many meanings. Our work is an effort to build clarity about what you mean when you discuss and address a patient's comfort." The audience calmed down . . . and our discussion proceeded in a lively but more open fashion thereafter.

I was pleased about the presentation and the subsequent discussion, and was hardly able to sleep that night because the experience was so stimulating. At 2 a.m., in fact, I had an "aha moment" which I remember clearly. For some reason, I woke up and the words of Orlando, an earlier nurse theorist, came back to me. I thought, "Comfort can be physical *and* mental!" I got out of bed and diagramed a two-dimensional, six-cell "comfort grid" with the three types of comfort (relief, ease, and renewal) across the top and the words "physical" and "mental" down the left side. In my mind, these six cells represented all the aspects of comfort.

Further Direction

Back at home, in a doctoral course on nursing concepts, I showed Professor Beverly Roberts my grid. "That's interesting," she said. "I have a new PhD grad coming to our class next week to discuss her work with a taxonomic structure (TS). I think your comfort grid is very similar to what she has done." Sure enough, when Margaret England presented her definition and rationale for a TS, I thought the comfort grid I had drawn fit the description. She stated, and Ray later elaborated, that a TS is a way to qualify or order its concepts for science. It is a classification system for concepts (such as comfort or suffering), species (such as plants or animals), things (such as rocks), or complicated systems (such as nursing diagnoses). This sounded promising!

I asked Margaret if I could meet with her after class and, when we did, she graciously looked at my grid and affirmed that, in her opinion, it was a TS. She pointed out, however, that "physical" and "mental" were not holistic—nursing had gone beyond that classification scheme. "You should look in the literature about holism and further delineate what holism really is," she said. She also suggested using the word "transcendence" instead of "renewal" because transcendence was already in the nursing vocabulary, thanks to the work of Paterson and Zderad (1976/1988).

FOUR CONTEXTS OF EXPERIENCE

The next year was spent looking at the nursing literature about holism. To do this, I delved into the literature, deciding in the process how to expand the TS to be truly holistic. From the simple physical and mental schema that I first envisioned, four contexts of human experience were explicated during a second literature review consuming yet another year. Those four contexts are as follows.

Physical Comfort

One thing was very clear to me as I began my exploration of the nursing literature on holism. I knew that physical comfort was the most obvious and agreed-upon context of comfort, and I had written previously of its complexity in my MSN assignment diagramming my practice. I wrote, "The physiological dimension addresses factors that affect the client's physical status, such as rest and relaxation, treatment of medical conditions, level of nutrition and hydration, and elimination of wastes" (Kolcaba, 1992a, p. 34). This broad usage of physical comfort was reinforced by introspection into my own physical comfort, and findings of nurse writers such as Joan Hamilton, Patricia Benner, and Marilyn Donahue. I encountered work from these scholars and others after I developed the full TS, and their views indicated to me that I was on the right track.

In what was a valuable study for reinforcing the TS, Hamilton interviewed 30 long-term care residents, 65 years of age and older. She asked the following four questions: (1) What is your definition of comfort? (2) What contributes to your comfort? (3) What detracts from your comfort? (4) How can you become more comfortable? (Hamilton, 1989). From the participants' responses, five comfort themes of equal weight emerged. I will relate these themes to the four contexts of experience in the TS. In tables further describing each theme, Hamilton included contributing factors, detracting factors, and proposed factors for more comfort which gave yet more insight into the holistic nature of comfort.

The first theme was comfort needs related to *disease process,* and the most prevalent detractor from comfort was pain. We would have expected this, but also on the participants' list of important contributing factors for physical comfort were regular bowel function, prevention or treatment of discomforts related to medical problems (such as leg or eye pain), and better diagnoses of the origins of such discomforts. Hamilton's findings, in the words of patients, supported my view that physical comfort encompassed all the physiological ramifications of medical problems, which *may or may not result in physical sensations* immediately. Examples of some necessary conditions for physical comfort, in this broad sense, are homeostatic mechanisms such as fluid/electrolyte

balance, stable and normal blood chemistries, adequate oxygen saturation, and other metabolic indicators of health. Abnormalities in any of
these physiological mechanisms must be treated (Relief) or kept at bay
(Ease) in order to maintain physical comfort.

An additional insight about physical comfort came from Hamilton's
(1989) comfort theme of *positioning*. Participants stated that sitting
correctly, having freedom to move independently in their chairs, good
positioning in well-fitting furniture, and being able to return to bed
when requested were central to their comfort. The importance of this
type of comfort was prominent in ergonomics and was associated with
increased function and productivity. Choice also was an important consideration. The definition of *physical comfort* that has evolved from Hamilton and later writers is "pertaining to bodily sensations and homeostatic
mechanisms that may or may not be related to specific diagnoses"
(Kolcaba, K., 1997).

Psychospiritual Comfort

Hamilton's (1989) second comfort theme was *self-esteem*, including faith
in God, being independent, feeling relaxed, being informed, and feeling useful. Here there was a blending of spiritual and psychological
comfort—a dilemma that I was encountering in my ongoing literature
review of holism. From this literature about holism, it was not possible
to differentiate the experiences of mind from those of the spirit and
of the emotions. For example, Howarth (1982) stated that the unifying
concepts within a holistic framework were physical, intellectual, and
spiritual, but the latter was in the generic sense, not related to religiosity.
There were wide definitions of spirituality that overlapped with conceptualizations of "mind" (Labun, 1988). Also encountered were wide definitions of spirituality that were operationalized by narrow empirical
indicators of religiosity (Reed, 1987). In addition, there were no specific
empirical indicators for transcendence, an important benefit of being
a spiritual person (Labun, 1988; Reed, 1987). It was for these reasons
that I combined the contexts of psychological and spiritual comfort
to form the psychospiritual context. *Psychospiritual comfort* combined
mental, emotional, and spiritual components of self. The definition
that has evolved is whatever gives life meaning for an individual and
entails self-esteem, self-concept, sexuality, and one's relationship to a
higher order or being (Kolcaba, K., 1997).

Environmental Comfort

Myra Levine (1967) proposed a model of holism based on the basic interaction of individuals with their environments (shades of Florence Nightingale). Similarly, Fuller (1978) said that the focus of nursing was the whole person in interactions with the environment. Wolanin and Phillips (1981) described a therapeutic milieu as being central for care of confused patients. Burkhardt (1989) also explicitly incorporated the environment into her model of holism. She stated that a holistic view "implies an understanding of the human person as unity where body, mind, spirit, and environment are descriptors of the interrelated manifestations of the person" (p. 60). Clearly, the right environment for healing and health promotion was considered an important source of comfort by nurses interested in holistic care.

Today, environmental comfort is a key aspect of units specifically designed to promote physical and cognitive function of hospitalized elders. These units are called ACE units, an acronym for Acute Care for Elders. Environmental aides such as handrails on the walls, nonglare lighting, calendars and clocks in rooms, high toilets with safety bars, minimal noise, and elder-friendly furniture are integrated throughout to maximize functional health (Panno, Kolcaba, & Holder, 2000). This type of unit is a perfect example of how environments of care can be manipulated to enhance comfort and function of patients.

The definition of *environmental comfort* that has evolved is "pertaining to external surroundings, conditions, and influences" (Kolcaba, K., 1997). Entailed in this definition is color, noise, light, ambience, temperature, views from windows, access to nature, and natural versus synthetic elements (Kolcaba, 1991).

Sociocultural Comfort

Participants in Hamilton's (1989) study stated that the friendliness and caring of all staff members was central in achieving social comfort. This included their approach and attitudes, continuity of care, and a meaningful schedule of events and activities. These elders also wanted to be better informed and more involved in their care, care planning, and decision making. Notable is the fact that they looked to their nurses and other personnel for their social comfort and did not mention the social support of their families as contributors to their comfort. In such instances, where patients have a limited network of support, nurses may be the most important source of social comfort and "therapeutic use of self" may enhance comfort more than nurses might realize.

This may be different today in acute and long-term care settings and/ or where "bare-bones" staffing is the norm. In these latter situations, a family member's presence is nearly a requirement for advocacy and safety. Nurses and other team members can facilitate social comfort of the family unit, however, by making them feel at home, important, intelligent, and valued.

Financial negotiations, conveying of information, and discharge planning occur in social contexts. Thus, these factors are considered to be elements of social comfort. When patients or their families need financial advice, nurses can make timely requests to social workers for assistance. When teaching patients/families about new regimens, it is necessary to inquire about financial burden associated with taking "designer meds." Whether with financial planning for medications or environmental aides such as handrails for the bathroom or the right wheelchair, nurses and/or social workers can help with referrals or assist with paperwork.

The definition of *sociocultural comfort* that has evolved is "pertaining to interpersonal, family, and societal relationships including finances, education, and support." Lately, the idea of culture has been added, to include family histories, traditions, language, clothes, and customs (Kolcaba, K., 1997). It may be important for the health care team to facilitate some of these customs during hospital stays or home health care to enhance social comfort.

THE TAXONOMIC STRUCTURE OF COMFORT

Juxtaposing three types of comfort (across the top) and four contexts of human experience (down the left), a 12-cell grid results, an expansion from the earlier 6-cell grid. The term renewal was changed to transcendence per Dr. England's suggestion, but the definition of that type of comfort remained the same. From the taxonomic structure and from qualities about aspects of comfort that were revealed in the literature reviews, a technical definition of *holistic comfort* has evolved: **Comfort is the immediate experience of being strengthened by having needs for relief, ease, and transcendence met in four contexts (physical, psychospiritual, social, and environmental)** (Kolcaba, 1997). It is this definition of comfort that I use throughout this book.

	RELIEF	EASE	TRANSCENDENCE
PHYSICAL			
PSYCHOSPIRITUAL			
ENVIRONMENTAL			
SOCIOCULTURAL			

Type of comfort:

Relief—the state of having a specific comfort need met.

Ease—the state of calm or contentment.

Transcendence—the state in which one can rise above problems or pain.

Context in which comfort occurs:

Physical—pertaining to bodily sensations, homeostatic mechanisms, immune function, etc.

Psychospiritual—pertaining to internal awareness of self, including esteem, identity, sexuality, meaning in one's life, and one's understood relationship to a higher order or being.

Environmental—pertaining to the external background of human experience (temperature, light, sound, odor, color, furniture, landscape, etc.)

Sociocultural—pertaining to interpersonal, family, and societal relationships (finances, teaching, health care personnel, etc.) Also to family traditions, rituals, and religious practices.

FIGURE 1.2 Taxonomic structure of comfort.

Kolcaba, K., & Fisher, E. (1996). A holistic perspective on comfort care as an advance directive. *Critical Care Nursing Quarterly, 18*(4), 66–76. (Adapted with permission of Aspen Publishers.)

In addition to a visualization of the content domain of holistic comfort, and a visualization about what the technical definition of comfort includes, the TS is useful for illustrating the following properties of comfort:

1. Comfort is an essential outcome for health care. It is patient focused—we are not talking about the nurses' comfort here although nurses' comfort is often enhanced when they know they have comforted patients effectively.
2. Comfort is a holistic and complex state and aspects of comfort are perceived simultaneously by recipients of care.
3. The aspects of comfort (each cell) are interrelated and attempts to target or measure them in a particularistic way are time consuming and inaccurate. However, a pattern of care can be established whereby patients' comfort needs are intuitively assessed in the four contexts.

By remembering the three types and four contexts of comfort, nurses and other team members can perform Comfort Care, not only in the sense of advance directives, but also in a proactive, healing, recovery sense. Comfort Care in any setting or population requires that patients' total comfort needs are assessed, interventions are designed to address comfort needs that have not been met by patients' existing support systems, and evaluation of the effectiveness of such interventions is carried out. Evaluations of interventions are done by comparing comfort scores before and after interventions are implemented.

When using the TS of comfort, differences between relief and ease are not terribly important except to remind us to attend to all known discomforts or risk factors for each patient in order to keep patients in a state of ease. Also, it is important to remember that, even when relief or ease cannot be achieved, we can intervene with comfort measures targeted toward transcendence in order to inspire or motivate patients to rise above their angst in order to do what must be done. This is very useful when patients must go through painful or unpleasant conditions associated with chemotherapy, rehabilitative therapies, or grief.

If a patient experiences comfort in every cell, or aspect, of comfort we can say that he or she is comfortable. However, such a state would be rare in stressful health care situations, where comfort needs are high. So the goal of health care is to enhance comfort compared to a previous baseline. This is the immediate altruistic outcome of a health care team that practices Comfort Care.

When doing an individual comfort assessment or intervention, it is most useful to address comfort needs in all four contexts (physical, psychospiritual, sociocultural, and environmental) with a single intervention or a series of interventions. For example, a simple back massage can enhance all four contexts of comfort, if the massage is accompanied by a warm, caring approach and preparation of the environment for relaxation. This leads to efficient patient care that is more satisfying to patients and nurses. As a guide for practice, education, and research the TS has survived the test of time (Kolcaba, 1991). Fortunately, it also is capable of evolving subtly over time as new insights and realities are generated in health care.

MUSINGS ON COMFORT QUOTE (CHAPTER 1)

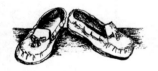

Comfort may be a blanket or breeze,
some ointment here to soothe my knees;
A listening ear to hear my woes,
a pair of footies to warm my toes;
A PRN medication to ease my pain,
someone to reassure me once again;
A call from my doctor, or even a friend,
a rabbi or priest as my life nears the end.
Comfort is whatever I perceive it to be,
a necessary thing defined only by me.
　　　　—S. D. Lawrence (student nurse)
　　　　(Kolcaba, 1995b, p. 289)

This poem was written by one of my clinical students after she used Comfort Theory for 8 weeks. Obviously, she related to this theory and understood its nuances for the patient and the nurse. I love the poem because it personifies individual preferences and needs for comfort measures, the importance of receiving the right comfort measure at the right time (no matter how insignificant it might seem), the essential ingredient of caring, and the central idea that comfort should be assessed from the patient's (or recipient's) perspective.

CHAPTER 2

The Mission

I hope that nurses will collectively move boldly into a future where knowing about, and doing something about human needs for comfort and relief from pain are clearly within nursing's realm.

—P. Chinn (1992, p. vii)

My mission is, and always was, to bring comfort back to the importance it held for nursing in the early years and to convince practicing nurses and other health care providers that they can and should provide Comfort Care. (Wouldn't it be wonderful if we were all on the same page?) From the time that I first applied the concept to my practice with Alzheimer's patients, and through the exploration phase, I was struck with the richness and complexity of the word. That very richness has positive implications for Comfort Care today, but the complexities call for a systematic approach to its use. I hope that this book builds the foundation and constructs the case to support my personal mission which began in nursing but which I now extend to the health care team.

The taxonomic structure (TS) of comfort identified the concept's many aspects and facilitated the technical definition of comfort (chapter 1). Although this definition was the first technical one of comfort, the concept was associated with health since the days of Nightingale. Indeed, in those earlier years, comfort was thought of as physical and mental, and interaction between physical and mental comfort and discomforts was acknowledged. As technology increased, this holistic but tacit understanding and valuing of patient comfort faded and comfort, for a time, was thought to be mostly an absence of specific discomforts. Therefore, for my present understanding of comfort, writings from the early years provided insight and confirmation that the origins of comfort in health care implied a more holistic meaning. To convey my understanding to you, I begin chapter 2 with a retrospective view of how comfort was used in nursing.

The last part of this chapter presents the views about comfort from contemporary nurses. When I began my work in the 1980s, I was not yet aware of the important work of Hamilton, Benner, Morse, and Donahue because their work had not yet been published. Indeed, at that time, I felt like a lone comfort pioneer because of the scant number of times I found anything about holistic comfort in the nursing literature. Later, I discovered that concurrent work was being done by several other nurses but in apparent isolation from each other. So, in the second part of this chapter, I summarize those articles that I discovered later, but nevertheless influenced or strengthened some of my current positions on comfort. This retrospective view covers the years from 1982 to 1992, when I began publishing what I thought were controversial articles about comfort. Chapter 2 ends with a summary of the insights gained from the entire review.

COMFORT AS A NURSING VALUE IN THE 1900s

In my quest for information about comfort in nursing, I wanted to determine if it had been defined at all in the early years, and if so, whether the definition was holistic. As early as 1859, Nightingale recognized that comfort was essential for patients. She said, "It must never be lost sight of what observation is for. It is not for the sake of piling up miscellaneous information or curious facts, but for the sake of saving life and increasing health and comfort" (Nightingale, 1859, p. 70). This was a general sense of comfort with no boundaries as to its meaning.

At the beginning of the 20th century, the term was used in a general sense as well. For example, Aikens (1908) stated that there was nothing concerning the comfort of the patient that was small enough to ignore. Comfort of the patient was the nurse's first and last consideration. A good nurse was one who made patients comfortable, and the provision of comfort was a primary determining factor of a nurse's ability and character. In 1926, Harmer stated that nursing care was concerned with providing a "general atmosphere of comfort" and that personal care of patients included attention to "happiness, comfort, and ease, physical and mental" (p. 25), in addition to rest and sleep, nutrition, cleanliness, and elimination. Goodnow (1935) devoted a chapter in her book, *The Technic of Nursing*, to "The Patient's Comfort." She wrote, "The nurse was judged by the ability to make her [sic] patient comfortable. Comfort was both physical and mental, and a nurse's responsibility did not end with physical care" (p. 95).

In this early period, patient comfort was highly valued by nurses who saw the provision of comfort as their unique mission (McIlveen & Morse, 1995). Comfort was important because cures were largely unavailable to physicians. Patient comfort was positive, achieved with the help of nurses, was nurturing, and, in some cases, indicated an improvement from a previous state or condition. Comfort resulted from physical, emotional, and environmental interventions and orders for specific comfort measures were under the physician's authority. Some common comfort orders in the period were for poultices, heat, and positioning of the bed.

Nurses were not to engage in health-related conversations with their patients because that was the job of the physician. Although emotional care was not one of the specified roles of nurses, physical comfort measures were acknowledged to bring about mental comfort of patients. In early nursing texts, the meaning of comfort was implicit, hidden in context, complex, and general. Many semantic variations, such as comforting, to comfort, in comfort, and comfortable were used, and the term could be verb, noun, adjective, or adverb, referring to either process or outcome.

Since that early time, the meaning and importance of comfort have undergone changes that parallel developments in health care. From its general meaning and significant worth in nursing at the beginning of the century, comfort evolved to a less important nursing value with a connotation more specific to the physical sense. Comfort was one of many strategies for promoting health and was secondary to other goals such as prevention of complications. In the 1950s, as analgesics became popular for pain control, few treatments for comfort were described (McIlveen & Morse, 1995). At this time, nurses took responsibility for patients' feelings, although nurses still couldn't talk about patients' medical conditions with them.

By the 1970s, nurses had more autonomy and could implement comfort measures without a doctor's order. Without doctors' orders for comfort, however, the motivation and recognition for enhancing comfort also diminished. In addition, as the presence of technology intensified, many traditional comfort measures were relegated to minor significance, were viewed as simple to administer, and were then implemented by assistive personnel. Anyone could provide comfort; therefore, comfort was no longer a specialized nursing goal nor included in definitions of skilled care. The term was still undefined in the discipline and semantically diverse, but now it was narrowly interpreted, written about rarely, and of course, not measured.

The 1980s saw many advances in medicine and cures from surgery, antibiotics, radiation therapy, and chemotherapy became more probable. Narcotics were used for treating severe pain. Comfort then became a secondary strategy for the larger purpose of effecting cure. Descriptions of comfort in nursing were limited and referred mostly to the physical state of the patient (McIlveen & Morse, 1995). The importance of family comfort began to emerge at this time and families were considered legitimate recipients of care and comfort measures (McIlveen & Morse, 1995). The interaction between the comfort of the patient and the comfort of the family was implied.

The connection in nursing literature between the comfort of patients and their being strengthened for rehabilitation was subtle but constant throughout nursing's history. Nightingale (1859) had claimed that patients who were kept comfortable by nurses would be in a better position to regain health. In 1931, Harmer noted a link between nursing comfort and the dictionary definition that included the component of strengthening. The linking of comfort, especially emotional comfort, to strength continued to be implied in the nursing literature through the 1980s (McIlveen & Morse, 1995). For example, a case study in a popular journal described how the nurse came to recognize that the patient's strength and courage to fight disease were derived from visits by his mother (Oerlemans, 1972). According to Paterson and Zderad (1976/ 1988), nurses helped their psychiatric patients achieve "more being" (an existential sense) in order to facilitate their function at highest possible levels.

In the 1980s, nurses promoted self-care, and comfort was a minor goal. Indeed, comfort was the *main* goal of nursing only when patients were terminally ill. It had been suggested previously that the goal of nursing reverted to comfort when there was no available cure (Glaser &

Strauss, 1965) and this trend was indicative of that observation. Also, where nursing settings were less under the control of technology, such as in hospice and long-term care, comfort was more important as a nursing goal. McIlveen and Morse (1995) suggested that this trend had broad implications for nursing in the 21st century, as demographics shift to large numbers of elders who wish for less technology and more comfort in their last months of life.

COLLECTIVE CONSCIOUSNESS: PRIOR RESEARCH AND THEORY

Knowledge development does not occur in a vacuum. Comfort seeds were planted in the early 1980s in apparent isolation, but they collectively enabled deeper understanding and theoretical growth. Ten years later, the time was ripe for comfort in nursing to be extended and promoted in new ways.

The review of groundwork that later supported or influenced my work begins in 1982, when Morse brought comfort to the attention of contemporary nursing, and will end with 1992, when I first operationalized the concept. The contributions of Morse; Benner; Rankin-Box; Donahue; Arrington and Walborn; Andrews and Chrzanowski; Hamilton; Gropper; and Neves-Arruda, Larson, and Meleis will be presented in this chapter in chronological order.

Morse (1983): *An Ethnoscientific Analysis of Comfort: A Preliminary Investigation*

A nurse who received her PhD in anthropology, Morse applied qualitative, "ethnoscientific" methods to begin the study of comforting actions of nurses. From careful observations and recordings came several phenomenological studies of nurses in different settings. Morse focused on the comforting actions of nurses and believed that these actions were central to nursing and must be thoroughly understood. The nursing actions Morse first described in her 1983 article consisted of touching and talking and, to a lesser extent, listening. Although she did not specify semantics of comfort, and often used the terms comfort, comforting, comfortable, and comforted interchangeably, she was describing the *process* of comforting within the context of nursing care.

The large body of qualitative work that Morse produced with her graduate students described the attributes of comforting nursing interactions with a variety of patients, such as those in a newborn nursery, emergency department, or medical-surgical unit. Her studies contained no intent to measure the comforting that occurred by the observed modalities of touch, listening, or verbal reassurance, nor did they propose a structure for enhancing patient comfort.

Morse's line of comfort research was very different from my line of inquiry that was launched a few years later with the diagram of my practice. My research focused on comfort as an outcome of specific comfort measures (interventions). It bothered me that both of us were producing work about the same concept and not addressing ways in which the two different approaches could be reconciled. Therefore, I went back to the philosophical approach, and asked my husband if there was an epistomological solution to my dilemma. A few days later, he referred me to the work of Dretske.

Process and Product Distinction

In 1988, the philosopher Fred Dretske made the important linguistic distinction between process and product when the term itself does not change. One example that he gave of such a term was *decay:* "The tree is decaying" (verb or process) and "The amount of decay (noun or product) is evident." The term *comfort* was another example: "The nurse comforts (verb or process) the patient" and "The patient's comfort (noun or product) is improved."

In ordinary conversation, terms such as decay and comfort usually are not confusing because common sense and context points to correct meanings. Dretske (1988), however, drew some distinctions between process and product that are important for addressing the semantic constructs of comfort. My understanding was that a process was a method of doing something, with all steps involved. Dretske, however, added the caveat that the process *specifies* the product. A product is the result of the process, or that which is produced. Because they correspond, comfort the process would *specify* the product of comfort as an end result. Unlike the word decay, however, comfort doesn't connote a true end product. Rather, enhanced comfort, compared with a previous baseline, is the desired outcome for the process of comfort. The important point here, though, is that the process does not occur as a separate entity from the product. The process is incomplete until the product, enhanced comfort, is brought into being. Second, the specified product signals an end or completion of the process. Individual events within the process are steps in bringing about the product. Third, the product subsequently can continue a causal series or be nested within a larger process. And fourth, the product is the destination of the process, so the product entails the rationale for the process (Dretske, 1988). Therefore, to study the process of comfort without evaluating the quality of the desired outcome of enhanced comfort is an incomplete exercise.

Comforting is a process when its corresponding product, enhanced comfort, is brought into being (Kolcaba, 1995a). Comforting can also be a process when the actions are intended to comfort even if intervening variables prevent the desired goal of enhanced comfort or if comfort is not being measured in such a way as to determine whether it was enhanced. Morse studied the process of comfort (actions of nurses) but not the product in her 20 years of comfort research. I studied the product of comfort (definition and measurement) but not the process in my first 10 years of comfort research (see chapter 3).

Morse and I approached the issues surrounding comfort from different perspectives and were then joined by others such as those included in this chapter. Collectively, we addressed the definition and description of patient comfort, factors that contributed to patient comfort, and measurement of the relative effectiveness of these factors. I worked hard to unify the work of other comfort scholars of whom I was aware, and in 1994 my Theory of Holistic Comfort for nursing was published (Kolcaba, 1994). This theory was utilized in the subsequent article incorporating Dretske's insights (Kolcaba, 1995a). In that article, the relationships were described between the descriptive work of Morse and my quantitative work with measurement. As Dretske had stated, only if comforting actions, or interventions, resulted in increased comfort, could they be considered successful. Thus, continual monitoring of patient comfort, with modification of the interventions as necessary, were required to ascertain when comfort had been enhanced. Morse's work supported and expanded upon the first part of my Theory of Comfort which stated that nurses provide comfort measures intended to address the needs of patients in stressful health care situations.

In my second 10 years of comfort work, I started looking at interventions to enhance comfort in different populations. I wanted to know if comfort could increase over time given an effective intervention, a phenomenon suggested by Murray (1938) and elaborated on in chapters 4 and 5. I proposed that the term "Comfort Care" include three components: (a) an appropriate and timely intervention, (b) a mode of delivery that projected caring and empathy, and (c) the intent to comfort (Kolcaba, 1995b). The term Comfort Care, therefore, included the work of Morse and myself. The term also was a proactive, interactive, and creative technique that went far beyond the rather negative connotation of comfort care as used in advance directives.

Benner (1984): *From Novice to Expert*

I first became acquainted with Benner's classic book when the College of Nursing at The University of Akron (Ohio), where I teach, adopted Benner's model for its curriculum. We used her nursing education model to develop competencies for our students and to describe our graduates. The fact that one of her expert skills included comfort gave credibility to my efforts at publicizing the importance of comfort as an outcome and to have students implement comfort care for their patients.

Benner included the provision of comfort measures under the "Helping Role" of nurses. She stated that the Helping Role "encompasses transformative changes in meanings and sometimes the courage to be with the patient, offering whatever comfort the situation allows" (1984, p. 49). She listed eight competencies entailed in the Helping Role: creating a climate for and establishing a commitment to healing, providing comfort measures and preserving personhood in the face of pain and extreme breakdown, presencing, maximizing the patient's participation and control in his or her recovery, interpreting kinds of pain and selecting appropriate strategies for pain management and control, providing comfort and communication through touch, providing emotional and informational support to patients' families, and guiding patients through emotional and developmental change. These competencies were interrelated, holistic, nontechnical, and significant for facilitating hope, recovery, and peace in patients. They represented the art of nursing and it was important for students to understand that the nontechnical skills (including comfort) were just as important, if not more important, to being an expert nurse than the technical skills students were so anxious to learn.

As an example, Benner described comfort during intubation that was provided through touch and communication. She interviewed a nurse expert who explained, "We would hold her hand and say, 'Everything is under control.' You just felt that was one of the most important things to do. Because [the patient] needs someone and she could only receive comfort and caring through touch and sight" (Benner, 1984, p. 64). Benner suggested that providing comfort through touch was symbolic of direct laying on of hands, "so central to nursing care" (p. 64). Intuitively, nurses literally have reached out as a way to demonstrate caring and provide comfort. Benner's voice also added to those of other contemporary nurses who sought to elevate comfort in nursing once again.

Rankin-Box (1986): *Comfort*

This British nurse observed in her short article that comfort relates to both physical and emotional well-being. But she cited the lack of any clear definition of comfort for nursing at that time and asked how we could interpret statements about the importance of comfort if we had no definition. For example, she used the statement, "An environment of optimum comfort enables the patient to progress more quickly and easily through the postoperative period." Clearly, comfort was important in this statement and comfort strengthened the patient. She asked, though, what is meant by the term and how can comfort be achieved in nursing care?

Also noted was the importance of providing care in an empathetic, caring way. Rankin-Box (1986) observed that there were many ways that nurses could deliver interventions, and that an intervention without a comforting delivery may not enhance a patient's comfort at all. Thus, she stated that providing comfort for patients was both an art and a science, as well as a process and outcome.

Rankin-Box also noticed the scarcity of articles about comfort when she was preparing hers. Most of the nursing literature was about management of discomforts such as pain, nausea, pressure sores, anxiety, or stress. She suggested that "nurses should ask not only what causes specific discomforts and how to alleviate them, but also what causes patients to feel comfortable and how do nurses maintain patients' comfort?" (1986, p. 340). Here she was using comfort as an outcome. Insights to answering these questions could come from introspection about our own experiences with comfort as well as conversations with patients.

Other insights from Rankin-Box were that (a) it was important for nurses to motivate patients to go through the trials of rehabilitation (corresponding to the type of comfort I called transcendence); and (b) there were physical, psychological, social, and environmental variables that nurses should assess and address as part of their comforting actions. Had I found her short article earlier, my search of the holism literature would have been much simpler! It was "comforting," however, to know that she agreed with me.

Donahue (1989): *Nursing: The Finest Art, Master Prints*

The purpose of this compilation of prints was to portray the "eloquent beauty of nursing and nursing care" (preface). Donahue selected master artworks to illustrate humanistic concepts prevalent in the discipline. In my opinion, this collection exemplified aesthetic and ethical knowledge in nursing. Through this medium, she explicated the essence of nursing, described its rewards, and elevated its mission. The concepts that she chose as examples of nursing art were: tenderness, skill, faithfulness, strength, love, care and caring, charity, spirit, excellence, dedication, discipline, tolerance, science, devotion, courage, innovation, concern, service, commitment, attention, trust, dignity, nurturance, professionalism, and comfort.

The painting entitled *The Red Cross of Comfort* was done by John Morton-Sale in 1939. It depicts a female with a large red cross on the long white pinafore covering her long blue flowing dress or uniform. From her dress and the title of the painting, we infer that she is a nurse tending a man with bandages on his eyes, specifically a Red Cross worker. Donahue spoke to the variety of environmental disasters in which these nurses "acted in the role of comforter." Improvising within a shattered environment, such as after floods, earthquakes, mine cave-ins, and epidemics, was an important part of nursing care.

Donahue's short essays about each concept were inspiring and informative. About comfort she wrote,

> This concept helps to create a world of nursing that encompasses the integration of concern for the spiritual, emotional, and physical aspects of patient care. It is through comfort and comfort measures that nurses provide strength, hope, solace, support, encouragement, and assistance to individuals, groups, and communities as they experience a multitude of life circumstances. (p. 27)

It was a thrill for me to find these words well after I had developed the taxonomic structure of comfort. These words validated my holistic conceptualization of comfort. Moreover, the image created by the picture and accompanying words captured my beliefs about what comfort is, how important it is to patients, and how central it is to nursing.

Arrington and Walborn (1989): *The Comfort Caregiver Concept*

In this article, a program is described that was initiated by a cancer patient named Mary. Mary requested that volunteer friends and acquaintances be scheduled by a coordinator if they wanted to help. The "comfort caregivers" came to her home every day for a few hours to assist in any way Mary wished. This program supplemented the regular skilled home care nursing services to which Mary was entitled.

When reading this article, the reality that nurses in home care or any setting can not get reimbursed for providing this type of comfort care troubled me greatly (and still does). When nurses feel the commitment to render comfort caregiving, they sometimes do so at risk of angering their employers because such activities may not be within the nurses' job description. Perhaps, in modern palliative care, these distinctions blur as comfort truly becomes the primary goal.

My understanding of holistic comfort was enriched further by thinking about what these comfort caregivers did. Their care consisted of helping with ambulation, screening phone calls, driving to doctors' appointments and out to the country, fixing meals, facilitating peaceful rest periods, listening to Mary's joys and frustrations, and sharing with Mary their own personal trials as well. These activities provided additional meaning for Mary who "felt comforted by the connection to the world of 'normal' activities" (Arrington & Walborn, 1989, p. 26). The caregivers ministered to the "whole person" (Mary's words) to provide "emotional support and contact with the outside world" and they provided "comfort and strength and helped Mary focus on healing and recovery" (p. 26). Too, comfort caregivers didn't necessarily have to be nurses.

Lastly, the authors reported that Mary was better able to cope with her daily problems and she remained more optimistic during her treatment and recovery process because of the added support (Arrington & Walborn, 1989). Here again was the connection between comfort and strengthening that had been prevalent in earlier nursing texts and in the semantic origins of the concept. So, while comfort was "nice" for nurses to facilitate, there was practical rationale for providing comfort as well. Namely, the strengthening properties of comfort produced better outcomes. In Mary's case, those outcomes were improved quality of life and feelings of control during a process that, otherwise, would have been more difficult.

Andrews and Chrzanowski (1990):
Maternal Position, Labor, and Comfort

This article was of initial interest to me because of the title. I was happy to see comfort in the title but, on the other hand, the title seemed an oxymoron from my experience 15 years earlier birthing my own children. I soon discovered, however, that these authors' idea of comfort was *not* holistic. (The idea of comfort during labor resurfaced in a more holistic way in the 21st century as discussed in chapter 6). But at the beginning of the 1990s, conceptualizations of patient comfort were still in a confusing state. For example, the authors stated that labor pain was related to a wide variety of psychosocial and physiological factors, yet the only one that was studied was maternal position. The Maternal Comfort Assessment Tool was used to estimate maternal comfort, but it was limited to measurements of the women's focus of attention, eye contact during contractions, muscle tension and activity during contractions, breathing pattern and vocal behavior, and verbalizations regarding ability to continue with labor. Information as to why these observable behaviors were inclusive or logical indicators of comfort was not given, and interestingly, the women were not asked about their comfort in any way. Also, no indicators of psychological comfort were included in the assessment, such as expressions of calmness, confidence, empowerment, or happy anticipation.

Findings were that women in the upright position had a significantly shorter maximum slope of labor than women who were lying down. Although mean comfort scores did not differ, upright women "appeared" to be more comfortable. In addition to the shorter labor, women in upright positions may have experienced beneficial psychological states during labor and birth, such as feelings of control and natural power of their bodies. These psychological aspects of comfort, which were not measured, might have made upright women more comfortable than women who were lying down.

A comment given at the end of the study was that women in upright labor positions may have been as physically uncomfortable as women in recumbent positions during the most intense phase of labor. However, the need for a holistic comfort instrument to measure psychological and physiological factors more accurately and directly in this population was apparent. Direct reports of comfort from the women themselves would have contributed clinical significance, and these reports could have been quantified with visual analogue scales or brief comfort questionnaires that were relevant to labor and delivery.

The idea, though, that comfort was complex, multidimensional, and holistic were reinforced by this early study. The need to measure comfort in a way that was congruent with clinical realities was also reinforced. Labor can be a transcendent experience given a certain type of empowering nursing care.

Hamilton (1989): *Comfort and the Hospitalized Chronically Ill*

When I saw Joan Hamilton's article announced on the front cover of *Journal of Gerontological* Nursing in June, 1989, I was filled with anxiety. I was sure my fledgling taxonomic structure would be redundant, inaccurate, trite, or overly objective. I soon realized that Hamilton's work complemented mine, however, as I had diagrammed the dimensions of comfort from my personal knowledge about comfort in Alzheimer's patients and two reviews of literature (see chapter 1). Hamilton, on the other hand, studied comfort from the patient's perspective using a predetermined interview format for data collection. Thus Hamilton humanized and enhanced my intuitive and academic approach. Best of all, Hamilton's work validated my library findings with descriptions of comfort from those who matter most—patients (see chapter 1). Her work provided ethical knowledge about patient comfort.

The five comfort themes that Hamilton discovered from her qualitative data supported my delineation of the contexts in which comfort was experienced in the following ways. First, she found that the theme of *disease process*, or physical comfort, consisted of more than the usual textbook emphasis on treatment of discomforts such as nausea and pain. Physical comfort also entailed, among other things, being able to go back to bed when requested, sitting correctly in furniture, and having regular elimination.

Second, Hamilton's findings that *furniture and personal belongings* could enhance comfort supported the environment as an important part of comfort. Moreover, the environment was something nurses could and should manipulate to enhance comfort and function, a mandate from Nightingale (1859) that had gotten lost amid the glamour of high-tech nursing. (In the 1980s, when a patient was disoriented in the

Intensive Care Unit, nurses used physical or chemical restraints to "manage" the patient until the patient "adapted" to the stressors of the unit.)

Third, Hamilton's comfort theme of *self-esteem* clearly fit into my category of psychospiritual comfort. Moreover, the subjects did not differentiate between psychological and spiritual comfort, because persons can be spiritual without going to church and vice versa. So combining these two contexts of comfort into psychospiritual comfort was supported.

Fourth, the comfort theme of *approach and attitudes of staff* supported the context of social comfort, and for Hamilton's residents in LTC, social comfort was dependent on the nursing staff. For example, empathetic and reliable nurses contributed to comfort, while inaccessible nurses and those who lacked understanding detracted from comfort. Additionally, residents wanted to be allowed to do things themselves, even if it took longer, and they wanted choices.

Fifth, Hamilton's findings hinted at the three types of comfort. *Relief* was discussed in terms of pain control and treatment for constipation. *Ease* was discussed in terms of keeping hospital life interesting, individualized, and flexible. *Transcendence* was discussed in terms of meaningful activities and caring relationships with staff. The residents described comfort in terms of its complexity and importance to their well-being. Moreover, they enjoyed talking about their comfort.

And sixth, while there was consensus among the residents that the five themes were equally central to comfort in their LTC facility, the residents also demonstrated individual preferences for ways nurses could contribute to comfort. At the end of the article, Hamilton stated, "The clear message is that comfort is multidimensional, meaning different things to different people" (Hamilton, 1989, p. 7). This statement was significant, as it voiced the importance of individualizing the process of comfort care.

Gropper (1992): *Promoting Health by Promoting Comfort*

Gropper stated that comfort was multidimensional and that persons integrated the physical, social, spiritual, psychological, and environmental dimensions of comfort in unique ways. She noted the strengthening component of comfort and said that when children were successfully comforted they were better able to use their energy for recovery rather than for expressing displeasure. When nurses deliberately comforted patients, they targeted expressed and unexpressed needs of patients in all dimensions. This included physiological needs such as functional elimination and oxygenation. Spiritual comforting offered by the provision of hope, was a "necessary component of the healing process" (p. 7).

An interesting point that Gropper raised, and which I have not seen since, is that in addition to conceptualizing comfort as a nursing action and nursing objective, comfort is a primary patient objective. She believed that for many, *health* was defined as physical and emotional comfort. She reasoned that most people sought health care when they felt discomfort or distress of one type or another. "Don't fix it if it ain't broke" was a popular motto in the early 1990s for people who were wary of entering the health care system.

Moreover, Gropper (1992) noted that people comforted themselves outside the health care system both in constructive and destructive ways. Therefore, a goal of nursing was to teach patients constructive ways to self-comfort. Constructive self-comforting activities included close family relationships, hobbies, healthy lifestyle choices, and engaging in meaningful activities. Destructive self-comforting activities included smoking, drug and alcohol abuse, gambling and other addictions, eating disorders, sexual promiscuity, and suicide. Considering these destructive behaviors as self-comforting activities was a creative idea, born of Gropper's observation that people first involved themselves with such behaviors because of their feelings of discomfort. If their discomforts were treated, needs for destructive behaviors would diminish and they would experience health.

Neves-Arruda, Larson, and Meleis (1992): *Comfort: Immigrant Hispanic Cancer Patients' Views*

Like some of the other work described above, the study by Neves-Arruda was a transcultural and qualitative study about comfort. Ten Hispanic cancer patients in a Texas hospital were asked, by a Spanish-speaking researcher, to describe comfort, list their comfort needs, and list their sources of comfort in their native language. Again the complexity of comfort was revealed, and many aspects of comfort in the Hispanic culture were very similar to those in the taxonomic structure (Kolcaba, 1991).

While most of the ideas about comfort were transcultural, some of the actual terms that were not easily translated into English provided further insight into the complexity of comfort. For example, Comodo was named by all participants and referred to accommodations, alignment, and positioning of body parts. Animo was used to describe the need to have a positive mental disposition, drive, or energy to be able to face what one was going through. Function and normalcy were especially important in the Hispanic culture. If patients could find the strength to maintain their normal routine, even while in pain, they stated that they were comfortable. "Being comfortable is living a normal life and not feeling like a sick person" (Neves-Arruda, Larson, & Meleis, 1992, p. 390).

All persons in the Hispanic sample agreed with previous samples across cultures that comfort could be provided by caregivers, friends, family members, self, and God. Nurses were important sources of social comfort. The patients in this study enjoyed talking about comfort, which also was true of other populations presented in this overview.

A new idea presented by Neves-Arruda was that the nature of health care situations affected the patients' expectations and needs for comfort. She believed, for example, that comfort needs in labor and delivery where the situation is desired and anticipated were less severe than comfort needs during cancer treatment. Patients with more rapid downward disease courses, and with more challenging symptoms, required more rigorous approaches to comfort than those with more chronic types of diseases. Thus the type of comfort given was determined by the prognosis of the health problem, in addition to the actual type and intensity of discomforts. The provision of meaningful, contextual comfort was presented as an additional challenge. Other recurring underlying themes were that (a) comfort is health, and (b) needs for comfort are universal. It was very apparent that comfort was important to patients in all of the above studies.

SUMMARY OF INSIGHTS

From the brief literature review above, several new insights or confirmations about comfort were found. Their influence will be apparent in the coming chapters. The insights were:

1. Comforting words and actions by nurses and other members of the health care team, as well as the intent to comfort, are important for interventions to be perceived as comfort measures by patients.

2. Comfort is a positive, dynamic state and the health care team can do more to enhance comfort if they go beyond the treatment of discomforts.
3. The strengthening properties of comfort produce better patient outcomes.
4. The measurement of comfort must incorporate its holistic nature.
5. The pattern of Comfort Care must be applied individually.
6. Comfort is important to all human beings.
7. Comfort-seeking behaviors can be constructive or destructive.
8. Health is comfort.
9. Comfort is contextual.
10. Expert nurses are proud of the ways in which they enhance patients' comfort. Their ability to do so, in part, makes them experts.
11. One way to enhance comfort is to manipulate the environment.
12. Comfort Care can be coordinated with other members of the health care team.

1992: COMFORT PERCOLATES TO THE TOP OF NURSING'S CONSCIOUSNESS

After 3 decades in nursing, during which comfort was minimized as a goal, a few nurses proposed that comfort be reinstated as a worthy nursing endeavor. In 1992, four nurse writers independently asserted that comfort was a crucial concept for nursing (Chinn, 1992; Gropper, 1992; Kolcaba, 1992a, 1992b; Morse, 1992). The nurse leader, Peggy Chinn, stated, "I wonder what nurse scholars might explore in our collective ideas and value systems to free any barriers to seriously developing the knowledge nurses need to provide comfort to others, or to alleviate human pain and suffering" (Chinn, 1992, p. vii). Morse made the argument that comfort, rather than caring, should be the focus of nursing care and that "the ultimate purpose of nursing is to promote comfort for the client rather than to care for the patient" (1992, p. 92). Gropper stated, "The traditional goal of nursing has always been to provide comfort, thereby relieving pain and distress, and restoring the health of the patient" (1992, p. 5). In the same year, without knowing about the others' work, I called comfort an important, nurse sensitive, measurable patient outcome that was essential for the patients' optimum function (Kolcaba, 1992b).

From these nursing articles, we see comfort reemerge as an important mission for health care. What's more important, Comfort Care was what patients wanted from their nurses. This change in focus occurred when I was operationalizing comfort as an outcome of patient care. To promote comfort required the administration of comfort measures in a caring way, while supporting the patient's own attempts to achieve comfort. Thus, caring was an essential component of patient comfort; and the patient would not be comfortable if the nurse acted in an uncaring manner.

MUSINGS ON COMFORT QUOTE (CHAPTER 2)

> I hope that nurses will collectively move boldly into a future where knowing about, and doing something about human needs for comfort and relief from pain are clearly within nursing's realm.
>
> —P. Chinn, 1992, p. vii

Here, Chinn pointed out that comfort is different from pain relief. She also spoke about the importance of comfort for patients and for fulfilling the mission of nursing. Most importantly, Chinn was concerned that her call for articles about comfort, for publication in the thematic nursing journal, *Advances in Nursing Science,* resulted in few submissions indicating, perhaps, a lack of interest prior to that time (1992), in patient comfort.

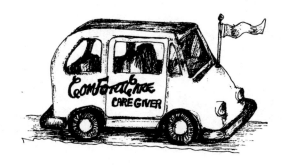

CHAPTER 3

Measuring Comfort

> If he paid for each day's comfort with the small change of his illusions, he grew daily to value the comfort more and set less store upon the coin.
> —Edith Wharton (1904), *The Descent of Man*, chapter 1

As discussed in chapter 1, the work on the taxonomic structure (TS) was completed about 1988. The process included two extensive literature reviews—one to develop the three types of comfort, and a second one to develop the four contexts of comfort. During those literature reviews, I did not discover other nurses doing work with comfort. The first article about the TS of comfort was finally published in late 1991 (Kolcaba, 1991).

In this chapter, I describe how I used the TS to develop the General Comfort Questionnaire (GCQ) and the issues I encountered while doing so. Then I share the agony and ecstasy of designing and implementing a dissertation study. Because my advisor, Dr. Roberts, was always several steps ahead of me, she wanted my study to be experimental. I was not ready to do this, but in the end, I compared the effects of guided imagery (a holistic intervention) on comfort (a holistic outcome) of women who did and did not receive the intervention. By sharing this process, readers may get "into my head," possibly enabling their future comfort studies to be generated more easily and more often.

DESIGNING THE FIRST COMFORT QUESTIONNAIRE

When I showed Dr. Roberts the final taxonomic structure with 12 cells, which was not yet ready to submit for publication, she asked quickly, "Can you design a questionnaire from that grid?" Confidently, I replied, "Yes, I think that would be easy." I still didn't know what she had in mind. My plan had been to publish the TS as a map of the content domain of comfort, and suggest to nurse researchers that they use it to design questionnaires that fit their specific setting. I was through with comfort, I thought . . . but Dr. Roberts had other ideas: "Why don't you design a comfort questionnaire—one that is general and that would be appropriate for persons in the hospital or at home? You can use the TS as a guide to create an equal number of items for each cell and an equal number of positive and negative items. I'd like to see it when you are finished."

In a few days, I had created the General Comfort Questionnaire (GCQ). It really was an easy task; deriving the TS had been the difficult and time consuming part for me. Dr. Roberts liked the questionnaire, but she wanted me to send it out to a panel of experts. I was taken aback: Who were the comfort experts? I was not aware of anyone, but computerized search engines were coming on the scene. Also, I was fortunate to have the dedicated and competent help of two reference librarians at The University of Akron, where I was teaching full time in the College of Nursing. They helped me find a comfort expert whose name was new to me. That expert was Janice Morse, who was just beginning to publish her qualitative articles about comfort.

Morse's first article about comfort was published in 1983 and, because it was not in a journal that was indexed at the time, I did not find it when I was doing my original literature review. (If I had come across it, my own work might have proceeded much differently or perhaps not at all.) When I read the article, I realized that our approaches to the exploration of comfort were very different. I was measuring comfort as an outcome; she was observing comforting actions of nurses. She was the only expert I could find at the time, however, so I mailed off my questionnaire with a blank TS. I asked Morse to identify the cell from which each of the 48 items had been derived, sort of the reverse of questionnaire generation.

I got a fairly prompt response from Morse. She sent back my stuff with the remark, "I don't know what you are doing." (Well, it *was* totally different from what she was doing.) That was the beginning and end of my contact with Morse. I did give the questionnaire to other nurses, though, including Joan Hamilton, whose article had just been published (1989). I asked about five experts, including Hamilton, if the 48-item questionnaire seemed to cover the content domain of comfort; I did not ask them to try to fit each question on the TS. I realized that asking experts to place the questions on the TS in the exact ways in which I had generated them was nearly impossible due to personal experience with comfort and interrelationships between cells in the TS. The results of this expert review were positive and I received encouragement and general agreement that the GCQ covered the content domain of comfort.

ISSUES TO RESOLVE ABOUT COMFORT

In designing my first comfort questionnaire, I had to clarify several issues for myself. The first was, "In what tense should these questions be stated?" Did I want patients who were answering the questionnaire to think back on their comfort or to have them answer according to how they felt about each item at the moment they were reading it? I thought about my own comfort and realized it was, for me at least, a very immediate state that could change rapidly. For example, I could be perfectly comfortable relaxing on my couch, watching a good TV show, when I receive a phone call from a daughter who is in distress. My comfort is shot—probably for the rest of the evening. Depending on how serious the distress, I may not feel totally comfortable for quite some time. Such, I thought, was the nature of comfort for patients, too. Later, I called this fragile quality of comfort "dynamic" and "state-specific." Therefore, all of the items in the GCQ should be in the present tense. Examples of items in the present tense were, "There are those I can count on for help" and "This view inspires me."

The second issue for me to resolve was, "Could one's perception of comfort be influenced by one's personality traits?" In my instrumentation class I learned about psychologist Charles Spielberger's work with anxiety. In the manual for using his state-trait anxiety inventory (STAI), which is now used widely in health care, Spielberger (1983) described how he initially developed an anxiety questionnaire of approximately 40 items. In the beginning stages of his work, he did not think about different types of anxiety. He then pilot tested his original questionnaire on hundreds of community dwelling persons, permitting him to do a factor analysis. This statistical procedure took all the responses, looked at how they clumped together (a rather mysterious operation for me), and produced factors or subscales.

After factor analyzing his responses, Spielberger found that his data clumped into two subscales: *state anxiety*, which is situational and likely to change quickly, and *trait anxiety*, which is an enduring personality characteristic and unlikely to change very much. This is an important distinction because a person with high trait anxiety would be likely to perceive everything more anxiously. From that time forward, his questionnaire was divided into two subscales. These subscales could be used singly or together, depending on the type of research (Spielberger, 1983).

I was familiar with this questionnaire and used it in some of my assignments in graduate school, which was how I happened to purchase the manual. The manual gave me a good background in instrument development and testing. It also caused me to ponder about comfort, "Does comfort have state-trait properties as well?"

To address this question, I referred to previous literature reviews and remembered that, in nursing, comfort could change very quickly and, early on, nurses believed part of their mission was to enhance comfort of their patients. Using those insights, I had defined comfort in part as being an immediate experience (Kolcaba, 1992b, p. 6). Therefore, I decided to limit my comfort questions to questions that were situational. This meant that *all* questions were state-specific, related to the present moment. The word comfort was not used in any of the questions to avoid response bias. Sample questions were, "I feel nauseated" or "I am hopeful." Respondents were asked to answer them quickly, according to the way they felt *at the moment*. Later, I discovered a statistical method for testing the state-trait distinction, and applied it to my dissertation data. Those results are reported in chapter 4.

The third issue was, "What should the tone of each question be?" I discovered in instrumentation class that questions should have a fairly neutral tone, allowing for a wide range of responses. For example, "I am able to walk around" speaks to a basic ability. If the question was written, "I am able to walk around easily," it would no longer be neutral.

The fourth issue was, "Should there be an even or uneven number of responses to each question?" I debated the fact that an even number of items forces participants to choose one side or another while an uneven number of items might produce many responses in the middle, either for lack of caring or lack of being able to decide. Therefore, the original GCQ was designed with four possible responses. There was no "middle of the road" choice.

The fifth issue was to choose the number of possible responses for each question. The number of responses is commonly 4, 5, or 6 in a Likert-type scale which I wanted to use. I had already ruled out 5 responses because that would offer a middle of the road choice. Six seemed like a lot of choices, so I opted for four; it also was the number Spielberger (1983) had chosen. Later, I would discover that more choices actually increased sensitivity while not having any negative consequences (at least in my comfort instruments), so I now recommend that all comfort questionnaires, even those for patients near end of life, contain six possible responses.

The sixth issue was scoring of the instrument. (This had to be decided before data collection began.) Therefore, I thought about what the numbered responses literally meant. If I assigned the highest response to strongly agree, because they were agreeing to positive statements about aspects of comfort ("I am able to walk"), then high scores would indicate high comfort. This was the semantic interpretation that I wanted. Thus the strongest, highest comfort state was indicated by the highest scores on comfort questionnaires from that time forward.

The seventh issue was to avoid compound statements in any question but, for me, that was easier said than done. An example of an early blooper, when I wrote some compound statements without realizing it, was the item: "My friends remember me with their cards and letters." This statement actually had two conditions. First, the respondent had to have some friends (family doesn't seem to qualify) and second, if the friends phoned but didn't send cards that wouldn't count. I learned through the expert panel review and a small pilot test which items were compound, because the respondents spoke up and told me that they were having a hard time answering those questions. Still, some compound statements slipped by as I discovered with the statistical item analyses.

The original GCQ that I showed Dr. Roberts went through several revisions as I learned more about instrumentation in my PhD program. How fortuitous it was that I had professors experienced in the difficult art of measurement. What I finally came up with is in Appendix A at the end of this book.

The specific cells in the TS from which each question was derived are indicated in Figure 3.1. I include this figure for anyone who thinks it might be helpful to see where I was coming from. A caution is also

	Relief *	Ease	Transcendence
Physical	14– 19– 48– 25–	1+ 36+ 20– 28–	15+ 29+ 5– 6–
Psychospiritual	44+ 46+ 22– 40–	2+ 7+ 31+ 38+ 24–	9+ 17+ 41– 45–
Environmental	3+ 27+ 12– 34–	11+ 47+ 32– 42–	30+ 33+ 18– 21– 35–
Sociocultural	37+ 8– 13– 26–	4+ 23+ 43+ 39–	10+ 16+

FIGURE 3.1   Plot of questions in the General Comfort Questionnaire on the taxonomic structure of comfort.

*Positive questions for relief often sound just like ease. Negative questions for relief designate needs that have not been met.

Note: It is permissible to have an unequal number of questions generated from each cell. Just make sure the content domain is sampled in each cell.

An equal number of positive and negative questions is used to prevent response bias, except in patients with diminished cognitive skills such as those near end of life.

Positive questions in the GCQ = 24
Negative questions in the GCQ = 24

included, though: Please don't try to duplicate the way in which I have diagrammed the items in each cell. I have found that once the questions are generated, they are interrelated and become part of the gestalt of holistic comfort. Other people have their own unique ideas about comfort and see the same questions a bit differently (we know that comfort is very individualistic). Also, it is difficult to discern between some questions under relief versus ease. That is because, once relief from a specific discomfort is achieved, the person will be in a state of ease. Worrying about these details will discourage you unnecessarily.

In spite of these ambiguities, the TS is very useful for making sure the content of comfort is covered. (I also call the TS a content map.) This is important when a researcher wants to adapt the GCQ. The TS is also useful for identifying which questions are in which subscale for subscale analysis. I was so pleased with the way the TS helped me construct the GCQ that I wrote it up for publication (Kolcaba, 1992b).

A Needed Boost

I submitted the article about the TS to *Image* and didn't hear back from the editor for about 9 months. I also presented the TS to MNRS in the spring of 1991. In the audience was Elaine Hogan-Miller, a clinical researcher who worked with cardiac patients. She wanted to test three methods for immobilizing patients' femoral sites after coronary angiography. One of the outcomes she wanted to measure, of course, was bleeding, but other patient-focused outcomes were difficult to identify. She described the experiences of her post-angiography patients: "They aren't in pain, but they are uncomfortable because of the immobilization. Their backs hurt, or their legs get restless, or they are bored." With this challenge in her mind, she came to hear my presentation on the TS of comfort.

After the presentation, Hogan-Miller approached me about comfort. She thought my definition of comfort was a good fit with her research population and I agreed. She thought, however, that the relatively short time frame that the patients were immobilized, about 6 hours, would not lend itself to measuring all aspects of comfort. So, over the telephone, we designed a questionnaire called the Physical Bedrest Comfort Measure, with 19 items relevant to the setting. An example was the item, "My muscles ache from being in one position" (Hogan-Miller, Rustad, Sendelbach, & Goldenberg, (1995). (For results of this study, see chapter 7.)

The reason I mention this study now is because that contact with Hogan-Miller incited me to ask the editors at *Image* about the status of my article. I wanted them to either publish my TS article or send it back to me so I could find another journal. I supported that request with the information that Hogan-Miller and I had just designed a second comfort instrument. I enclosed a copy of her correspondence about our comfort questionnaire for post-cardiac angiography patients. This bit of evidence got the article accepted in record time and it was published 6 months later (Kolcaba, 1991).

The other positive experience with this study was the convenient congruence between holistic comfort and patient immobilization. Here was a population which demonstrated that comfort was more than absence of pain because patients could be very uncomfortable and have no pain. I was encouraged that comfort questionnaires would be useful for nurse researchers in other unique types of settings (I wasn't sure where).

PILOT TEST OF GENERAL COMFORT QUESTIONNAIRE (GCQ)

"Does anyone want to do a pilot test? It will really help you when you get ready to graduate." I should have been suspicious when I was the only student in the class to raise a hand! In retrospect, I have a feeling as well that Dr. Roberts directed the question to me, although the thought did not cross my mind at the time.

So, I talked to Dr. Roberts about what a pilot test would entail. I had recently shown her the 48 questions of the GCQ, and she wanted me to do a psychometric study of the instrument. I didn't know what she meant. She explained that I would get a heterogenous group of patients and community dwelling persons to answer the questionnaire one time. Then I would get a reliability score, including item analyses, and do a factor analysis. I still didn't know what she meant. This was how one tested a new instrument, which was what I had created with the GCQ.

"How many patients would I need?" I asked naïvely, not having done any previous data collection.

"Well, factor analyses requires 10 subjects per question, so 480 subjects . . . " Now I was naïve, but not stupid. That number sounded very high.

"480?"

"Well, you could do data collection in several sites." (I didn't know that each site required its own Institutional Review Board [IRB] process.)

"OK, I guess I could do that over the summer." I still can't believe it. You can tell by my comments that I had so much to learn—writing a proposal, informed consent, IRB applications, finding and keeping good data collectors, presenting the project to gate keepers, et cetera.

Yes, I learned a lot. No, it did not help me graduate; it actually slowed me by at least 2 years. Nor was I permitted to use this study for my dissertation.

Did I get 480 subjects? No, after 1 1/2 years of data collection, and 256 completed questionnaires, I became proactive and practical. I found a citation in a research text that said five subjects per question was sufficient for factor analysis (Tabachnick & Fidell, 1989, p. 603). I showed it to Dr. Roberts who let me off the hook, and I began data analysis.

Am I glad I did it? Yes! Obtaining the psychometric properties, including the factor analysis, for the GCQ proved to be the evidence that would support the rest of my comfort career.

Psychometric Properties of the GCQ

To my surprise, the Cronbach's alpha was .88, very high for a new instrument (Kolcaba, 1992b). Perhaps working from a theoretically driven TS worked, I thought. Factor analysis was a difficult proposition for me, although I was doing it while enrolled in Dr. Youngblut's instrumentation class mentioned earlier. In that class I learned the theoretical reasons for doing one type of rotation versus another type, asking the computer for a specified number of factors versus letting the computer choose, and how to interpret the findings. But the factors were not turning out as I thought they would. That is, I thought the items would load on the four contexts of comfort (physical, psychospiritual, social, and environmental) because these were so much easier to explain and differentiate than the three types of comfort (Relief, Ease, and Transcendence). Therefore, I kept asking my statistician friend to try different rotations on her university's mainframe (a major financial cost), with all kinds of combinations of forced factors.

I was literally in the middle of all this, when I received galleys from *Advances in Nursing Science*. This was my manuscript about how to operationalize comfort using the recently published TS. Unfortunately, the publisher wanted me to add any information I had about the psychometric properties of the instrument. For reports on the factor analysis, I did not have the help of the editors nor my professor at the time because the galleys were due back immediately. To this day, I am not happy with the way I hurriedly put together the results for that article (Kolcaba, 1992b); this chapter gives me a chance to report those findings more accurately. Incidentally, all of the different rotations achieved approximately the same result, a fact that took me a long time to see.

If I could indeed rewrite page 8 of the article entitled *Holistic Comfort: Operationalizing the Construct as a Nurse-Sensitive Outcome* (Kolcaba, 1992b), this is what it would say (you need not have the article in front of you to "get my drift"): "Initially, the Principal Components Analysis, varimax rotation, extracted 13 factors with eigenvalues above 1.0. The 13th factor had only one item and was collapsed into one of the other factors that was semantically similar. Therefore, this result was consistent with the 12-cell taxonomic structure. In addition, factors clumped together in three subscales on the scree plot and semantically were similar to the *Types of Comfort (Relief, Ease, and Transcendence)*. This loading accounted for 63.4% of the variance in the 48 items."

In the article, at the bottom of page 8, I list reliabilities of revised subscales, which were achieved by deleting weak items and rerunning the item analysis. However, I did not retest the revised instrument with a subsequent population. Therefore, these reliabilities are only guidelines for possible ranges of Cronbach's alphas for the subscales. Note that reliabilities ranging from .66 to .80 for the subscales are lower than for the whole GCQ (.88). This is because lower numbers of items generally decrease reliability scores.

I want to explain why the table on page 7 of that article has different labels than my web pages and later articles such as *A Holistic Perspective on Comfort Care as an Advance Directive* (Kolcaba & Fisher, 1996). While first contemplating the meaning of the Factor Analysis (FA), it appeared that subjects responded to the GCQ items based on intensity of comfort needs. Their needs for Relief were the most pressing and therefore, I thought that the subscales, Relief, Ease, and Transcendence may be on a continuum. Since that time, I prefer to think of the three subscales as being different from each other, particularly transcendence. This way of thinking is consistent with patients having some needs for relief partially met, and still having needs for transcendence over the needs that couldn't be met. For example, laboring moms can be in momentary ease, as in between contractions, but still require transcendence to buoy them for the next contraction. Ease and relief are also quite different, because relief entails a prior discomfort that was relieved, while ease can stand alone. For these reasons, I later changed the label for the subscales from *Intensity of Unmet/Met Comfort Needs* to *Types of Comfort*. I use Types of Comfort throughout this book.

Likewise, the heading *Internal/External Needs* was changed to *Contexts in Which Comfort Occurs*, because I no longer believe that the contexts in which comfort is experienced represent a continuum like the label in the 1992a article implies. The numbers on the grid, designating a cell from a particular row and a particular column, can be disregarded. They proved to be more trouble than they were worth.

The GCQ did show statistically significant sensitivity in expected directions between several groups of respondents (construct validity).

The early descriptions of group differences were (a) the community group (30 subjects) had higher comfort than the hospital group, and (b) people with higher comfort demonstrated higher estimates of their own progress in rehabilitation.

I think it's important to discuss here how my closed mind influenced the process of the FA. First of all, I was not confident that I would have a coherent factor structure, as my questionnaire was homespun, by a quite ordinary person (me). *If* the data were so cooperative as to produce a coherent structure, I was sure the items would load on four factors (contexts) rather than three factors (types of comfort). I was so sure, in fact, that I tried every conceivable rotation to make that happen. It didn't work. Finally, I looked at the *wording* of the items and their placement on the TS. I saw then what I should have seen much earlier, if I had been more objective. What I saw was that the items loaded on the three types of comfort, not the contexts. I was angry at myself for wasting so much time and money, but happy that the GCQ had a factor structure that was congruent with the TS after all.

Post Publication

Since the publication of that article, many nurses have written to me asking for a copy of the GCQ. Although I had discussed the "revised" GCQ in the article, hypothetically removing weak items, most correspondents wanted the original 48-item questionnaire. They wanted to see all of the original items, and delete ones that weren't relevant for their research questions. Then they could "fill in the blanks" on the TS with their own items. I support this approach wholeheartedly, hoping that nurses will come forward from a myriad of nursing settings and with unique patient problems in which comfort is an appropriate outcome.

Since that publication in 1992, many requests for the GCQ have come, in the earlier years by snail mail and later by e-mail. Most often e-mail contacts are made through my web pages (The Comfort Line) which are linked to the Nursing Theory Web Page (Kolcaba, K., 1997). Some of the settings in which nurses have been interested in measuring patient comfort include a burn unit, gynecological examination, hospital ship, medical and surgical, midwifery, hospice, long-term care, radiation therapy, immobilization, infertility, acute care for elders (ACE), urinary incontinence, newborn nursery, emergency department, psychiatry, and critical care. These settings are where comfort needs are very complex and where the outcome of patient comfort is so much more than the absence of pain.

Now, researchers who find my Web pages can download the GCQ with instructions for adapting it to any given population. (It is also included in Appendix A of this book.) I try to answer all e-mail questions, and I arrange phone conferences in my efforts to promote patient comfort as a value in nursing. Usually, although I would like it, I don't receive feedback after these initial contacts. I am hopeful that this drop off will change as we all realize the benefits of working together.

DISSERTATION TIME

"For your dissertation, I want you to do an experimental study." That was an out-of-the-blue comment by Dr. Roberts, who as I said, was always a few steps ahead of me. By that time, I knew what an experimental design entailed: namely, a lot of work! I wondered, among what population could I expect to find a positive and timely change in comfort, given an effective intervention? That question would haunt me for the next year.

The other major challenge in my life at the time was my brother's terminal diagnosis of malignant melanoma. He was 43 years old, 18 months younger than I, and my only sibling. John and I were close, but he approached his cancer differently than I would have and rarely asked for my advice (now that's hard for us nurses!). John tried every known cancer treatment in the effort to prolong his life. Still, his condition and quality of life deteriorated, and his days in the hospital where I worked PRN were more numerous. I became acquainted with the world of oncology nursing, and most of what I saw inspired me. These nurses knew the importance of patient comfort, and I grew more interested in pursuing the holistic comfort of cancer patients. I also thought that I could demonstrate a change in comfort more easily in an oncology setting, because the patients' comfort needs were extremely acute yet often amenable to mind-body interventions. Thus, for my dissertation, I strayed from my gerontological roots where, I thought, comfort needs were so chronic that I might not be able to demonstrate a change over time and still graduate in time to have a meaningful research career.

Gradually the idea for my dissertation took shape: I would develop a guided imagery (GI) audiotape for women with breast cancer going through conservative treatment. Breast conserving therapy consisted of lumpectomy and radiation therapy (RT). My *research* question was: Will women who receive GI while going through RT for early-stage breast cancer have greater comfort over time compared to a control group? My *real* question was: Can I demonstrate a change in comfort over time in persons who receive an effective and repetitious intervention? I was hoping, even though comfort was a dynamic state and could change quickly, that a trend of increasing comfort could be established empirically.

The audiotape medium enabled me to deliver the same message over and over to all women in the treatment group. In the script for GI, I built in positive statements regarding every cell in the TS of comfort known to be important for this population. To write the script for the audiotape, I returned to the literature—this time regarding breast cancer and RT. I found an excellent recording artist who specialized in GI. I made sure to cover the content domain of comfort by working with the TS and the questions I had developed for each aspect of comfort. I received help from the RT nurses, technicians, and physicians to fine-tune the tape and design of the study. The women were asked to listen to the tape at least once every day, at their convenience, with tape players that the study provided. This way, the protocol as well as the message were consistent.

To adapt the GCQ to women with breast cancer, I deleted questions that were not relevant for my new setting. The remaining questions were plotted on a blank TS, which then gave me a picture of what aspects of comfort I had to address in my questionnaire in order to cover the content of comfort. The literature pinpointed critical comfort needs specific to this population. From this appreciation of needs, I developed positive and negative questions to complete and balance the TS for this population. I also had the help of RT nurses, physicians, and patients in developing all parts of this study.

A consideration when developing the Radiation Therapy Comfort Questionnaire (RTCQ) was the length of time it would take for the women to answer it. The nurses thought, and it was later confirmed, that many research participants would choose to meet me in the RT department rather than in their homes, at least after the first meeting. So, the design of the study was to administer all questionnaires immediately prior to RT and this would be done three times: (1) Before simulation and RT started, (2) three weeks into RT, and (3) three weeks after RT was completed. A 48-item questionnaire was deemed too long by the RT staff, and probably too stressful for the women. (This issue arises frequently but it has been our experience that 48 questions [4 from each cell], creates a questionnaire that is manageable, well-balanced, and has high reliabilities.) However, for this study I used a 26-item Radiation Therapy Comfort Questionnaire (RTCQ). The RTCQ was pilot tested with more patients, along with the GI tape, and I was in business.

I also developed, for the first time, visual analog scales (VASs) to measure the three subscales of comfort (Relief, Ease, and Transcendence). These subscales emerged from the factor analysis in the psychometric study of the GCQ (Kolcaba, 1992b). My stems for the VASs were, "I have many discomforts right now" (Relief), "I am feeling at ease right now" (Ease), and "I am feeling motivated, determined, and strengthened right now" (Transcendence). I developed the VASs, in part, to begin to establish concurrent validity for comfort. There were no other measures available for comfort. Secondly, I wanted to see if VASs could measure patient comfort more efficiently than the longer questionnaire. This might have clinical significance both for this population and down the road. The RTCQ and VASs are in Appendixes B and C respectively.

The study went well. Two RT departments at teaching hospitals in nearby cities agreed to let me collect data at their sites. When we did our pilot test, we asked specifically if there was anything we forgot to ask in the questionnaire, anything we forgot to say or did not say well in the audiotape, and whether the instruments were easy to use. When everyone was satisfied with the protocol, the tape and tape player, the instruments, and IRB approvals were in place, we proceeded. The outside member of my dissertation committee was a radiation oncology physician.

Nurses told the women about the study during their first visit to the RT department. When the patients first heard about the study, about half the women burst into tears (another reminder that they really had breast cancer); the other half wanted to enroll. The nurses faxed to my home the names and phone numbers of those who wanted to enroll, and upon arriving home I called the women immediately in order to see them before their simulation visit. This required much juggling of my schedule and was very stressful for both me and the women. As buffers to the stress, I had some wonderful student helpers. The women were also wonderful, and they really liked the tape. We collected complete data sets (three visits for each woman) on 53 women, which took a year after IRB approvals were obtained (Kolcaba & Fox, 1999). I am greatly indebted to the personnel and my students for helping me with data collection.

Another issue that took a great deal of time to sort out was the method for data analysis. I had consulted with not only my statistician friend, Dr. Christine Fox, but also with Dr. Richard Steiner, Department of Statistics at The University of Akron. We agreed on Repeated Measures Multivariate Analyses of Covariance (RM MANCOVA), with the covariate being baseline state anxiety (Spielberger, 1983). Other possible covariates could be any baseline group differences we detected from demographic data.

I like the test statistic MANCOVA because it is "holistic." It looks at group differences, over time, and the interaction effects between time and group. Also, baseline data serve as each subject's own control. When the test statistic is significant, post hoc tests determine which group has the best outcome (in this case, comfort). By looking at all of these factors at one time, I believe RM MANCOVA truly captures the essence of a holistic study design (Kolcaba, 1998). Also, I use an alpha of .10 for significance if my interventions have no negative side effects (Lipsey, 1990).

Results

By the time my data were collected, Christine Fox had moved to a different university about 150 miles away. E-mail was just coming on the scene, but it was not sophisticated enough to send attachments. Therefore, most of the detailed work required for analyses was done by phone, snail mail, or fax. The phone conversation that I remember distinctly went as follows:

"Hi Christine." (Small talk.) "Have you gotten any results yet with my data?"

"I'm working on it right now. Just a minute." (Clicking of computer keyboard in background.) "Well . . . you have a significant difference between groups." (I screamed!)

"But which group is higher on comfort?" (My first post hoc test and a few more agonizing minutes of computer keyboard clicking.)

"The treatment group is higher." (Christine's communication style always had been understatement.)

Shouts of joy from me, and disbelief, relief, visions of graduation danced in my head. I have always been emotional, but this was an exciting day. I had demonstrated that comfort could be measured with enough sensitivity (strength of the instrument) to detect a change in the state of comfort over time given an effective intervention ($p = .07$ for differences between groups over time). The instrument performed well with a Cronbach's alpha of .76 ($n = 53$, 26 questions). Finishing my dissertation entailed the usual ups and downs (described in more detail in chapter 5), but I graduated about 9 months after data collection was completed. I was in the PhD program for 10 years and when I graduated I was 52 years old and a grandmother.

While I was happy with the statistical performance of the RTCQ, the performance of the VASs was mixed and required more involved secondary analyses later. Hence, these scales were not discussed in my first dissertation article (Kolcaba & Fox, 1999). The Total Comfort (TC) Line was not sensitive to differences in comfort over time ($p = .82$). The scores for Summed Comfort Subscales (Relief, Ease, and Transcendence) provided data that were nearly significant ($p = .17$) and seemed to be more sensitive to individual perceptions of comfort. These findings suggest that asking patients to rate their total comfort on a scale of 0–10 covers too many attributes about individual comfort. That is, factoring in differences in meaning and emphasis between subjects results in evening out the responses. In clinical settings, however, I believe that asking a patient to rate his/her comfort from 0–10 will result in meaningful conversations about detractors from comfort, so that the nurse knows how to proceed with Comfort Care. A complete discussion of the properties of the four VASs is presented in chapter 4 and in Kolcaba and Steiner (2000).

Correlations between the VASs and the RTCQ supported preliminary concurrent validity between the two measures of comfort. Concurrent validity is the extent to which a measure correlates with another simultaneously obtained measure of the same trait or state (Goodwin & Goodwin, 1991). Because there was no gold standard for measuring comfort in this population, correlations between the VAS for total comfort and the RTCQ were computed. We believed that the RTCQ would demonstrate a medium to strong positive correlation with the VAS for total comfort because both instruments were designed to measure holistic comfort and both were administered at the same three time points to the same research participants. Data were skewed to the right because most women indicated relatively high comfort on the VASs (7.3 on scale of 1–10, with 10 being high comfort) and in a rather narrow range (standard deviation 1.58). Thus, non-parametric measures of association were performed. Pairwise correlations between the RTCQ and the VAS for total comfort revealed moderate correlations at each of the three time points: Time 1 = .31, $p = .02$; Time 2 = .31, $p = .02$; and Time 3 = .44, $p = .00$. We concluded there was moderate concurrent validity between the two comfort instruments (Kolcaba & Steiner, 2000).

SUGGESTED METHODS FOR COMFORT STUDIES (KOLCABA, 1997)

I make the following recommendations about methods on my Web site, entitled The Comfort Line, to all my contacts who are interested in doing a comfort study:

1. A comfort study has a good chance of demonstrating significant differences in groups if the intervention (developed with the TS) is congruent with the outcome (also designed with the TS). Holistic interventions, such as music or art therapy, GI, massage, therapeutic touch, and cognitive strategies can be targeted to every aspect of comfort in the TS. Thus, the intervention and outcome are congruent.

2. Gather data over time, with at least three measurement points, including one baseline measure. This part of the design is holistic because it looks at the entire experience of the research participants.

3. Consider using an alpha of .10, a recommendation of Lipsey (1990), who believes that, when interventions have few side effects, social scientists (and nurses) incur greater risk of Type II error while protecting aggressively for Type I error. (Type I error is the possibility of finding significance when that finding would be incorrect; Type II error is the possibility of failing to find significance when that finding would be incorrect.) In other words, with the stringent selection of alpha of .05, we often miss finding significance when the intervention really *is* associated with positive effects. Many of our holistic interventions, which have no known side effects, would not have significant findings at the more stringent alpha, but would be declared effective at an alpha of .10. With interventions that have side effects, however, such as new drug protocols, alpha of .05 or .01 is still recommended.

4. If the MANCOVA is significant, the first post-hoc question you will ask is, "Which group has the highest level of comfort?" When you test assumptions for MANCOVA, you do T-tests at each time point, which tell you which group is highest. So, really, this question has already been answered—you just need to put the information together.

Your second post hoc test can be a trend analysis that reveals the slope of improvement—whether it is linear, curvilinear, quadratic, et cetera (Stevens, 1992). A linear relationship between groups, with the treatment group showing steadily increasing comfort while the comparison group stays about the same at three time points, is a great outcome, consistent with the theory (see chapter 5).

If you are thinking about doing a comfort study, it may not be necessary to develop your own instrument. In fact, as I have related, doing so is difficult and time consuming. There are several other comfort instruments available that were designed by others or you can adapt the GCQ to fit your needs. For readers to have an overview of what has been done and how various empirical comfort measures have performed, Table 3.1 is provided.

MEASURING COMFORT IN YOUR OWN POPULATION

Because the measurement of comfort is relatively new, there are many populations and research problems where comfort instruments have not yet been developed. I hope this will not deter any researchers from adapting the GCQ for their own purposes. For example, one group of hospice nurses wanted to shorten the Hospice Comfort Questionnaire (HCQ), and spent some time tallying votes from 14 experts on questions that should be retained (25 items) and those that could be deleted. (Our item analysis of the 49 items on the HCQ revealed that all items were equally strong for nearly 100 patients over Phases I and II. Thus there was no statistical direction for shortening the 48-item instrument.) Also, our sample of nearly 100 patients [over Phases I and II] had no difficulty with the length of the instrument but they only answered it one time [Novak, Kolcaba, Steiner, & Dowd, 2001].)

When adapting the GCQ, I would caution you to do a small pilot study of the instrument with representatives of your target population, to determine the reliability coefficient (Cronbach's alpha) for the revised instrument. A caution here is that a shortened questionnaire probably will have a lower reliability score.

Adapting the General Comfort Questionnaire to Your Population (Kolcaba, 1997)

1.   Delete questions from the original GCQ that are not relevant for your population.
2.   Place the number of retained questions on the TS of comfort, noting whether they are positive or negative. This process creates a map of the questions you presently have in the content domain of comfort. (Please remember to cite the origin of the taxonomic structure in your proposals/articles, e.g., Kolcaba, K. [1991].) You can also cite

TABLE 3.1 Psychometric Properties of Existing Quantitative Comfort Instruments

Name of Instrument	Reliability	No. of Items	No. of Subjects	Structure Analysis?	Reference
Maternal Comfort Assessment Tool (observer rating)	Interrater: 89%	7	40	NA	Andrews & Chrzanowski, 1990
Dementia Comfort Checklist (observer rating)	Correlation Coefficient r .88	9	82	NA	Hurley et al., 1992
General Comfort Questionnaire (GCQ) (patient rating)**	Cronbach's alpha .88	48	256	Factor Anal.: Relief, Ease, Trans.	Kolcaba, 1992b
The Comfort Scale (Distress in Pediatric Intensive Care Units)	Interrater: .84 Int. Consis.: .90	8 and VAS	50	Correlations between 8 dimensions	Ambuel, Hamlett, Marx, & Blumer, 1992
Physical Bedrest Comfort Measure (patient rating)	Cronbach's alpha .73	19	30	No (not enough subjects)	Hogan-Miller et al., 1995

(continued)

TABLE 3.1 *(continued)*

Name of Instrument	Reliability	No. of Items	No. of Subjects	Structure Analysis?	Reference
Radiation Therapy Comfort (position of bed)	Sig. Diff. Bet. Groups	1 VAS	17	No	Cox, 1996
Comfort Questionnaire (dehydration/hydration at end of life)	NA	14-pt. Likert scale	31	No	Vullo-Navich et al., 1998
Radiation Therapy Comfort Questionnaire (RTCQ) (patient rating)**	Cronbach's alpha .76	26 and VASs	53	No (not enough subjects)	Kolcaba & Fox, 1999; Kolcaba & Steiner, 2000
Urinary Incontinence and Frequency Comfort Questionnaire (UIFCQ)* (patient rating)	Cronbach's Alpha .82	23	40	No (not enough subjects)	Dowd, Kolcaba, & Steiner, 2000
Infant Comfort Behavior (Pain)	Kappa .63–.93	6 and VAS	158	LISREL	Van Dijk et al., 2000
Hospice Comfort Questionnaires (HCQ)* (patient and caregiver rating of their own comfort)	Cronbach's alpha Patient .98 Caregiver .97 VASs	48 48	48 38	No (not enough subjects)	Novak et al., 2001

*Instruments reprinted in article.
**Instruments available through Web site: *www.uakron.edu/comfort/comfort_theory.html.*
Reliability for visual analog scales (VASs) determined by test-retest and reported in chapter 4.

the psychometric properties of the original GCQ (Kolcaba, 1992b) when presenting your plans for an adapted instrument. Just indicate that they provide your adapted instrument with preliminary validity and reliability.

3.   Fill in the map with your own positive and negative items that are specific to your population and/or research problem. You want to achieve a balance across the entire content domain of comfort. If you decide that one of the contexts or types of comfort is not important to assess for your population/problem, take that row or column out, but justify the exclusion in your write-up.

4.   When constructing your questionnaire, it may be difficult to discern between positive questions for relief and ease. I think of the difference as this: relief is the immediate lifting of an existing, acute discomfort, while ease is a longer lasting and positive condition such as contentment, peacefulness, or restfulness, that connotes a possible predisposition to a discomfort. To keep a patient in a state of ease, however, the health care team should be aware of the acute discomforts to which he or she is predisposed.

5.   Scoring is done by reverse coding the negative items and adding the total. Higher scores indicate higher comfort. You can also create scores for each subscale (Relief, Ease, and Transcendence) using your map of the content to delineate which items belong to which subscale.

6.   My husband, a professor of philosophy, has published an article about persons being in and surrounded by their environments (Kolcaba, R., 1997). My comfort instruments are congruent with his views, and therefore my sense of environment presently includes those features external to persons like noise, light, and furniture. This definition explicates the necessity of the health care team to manipulate surrounding environmental features to enhance patient comfort. This is also Nightingale's view of the environment.

Persons and groups of persons including health professionals possess their own energy fields. While my comfort instruments currently do not measure persons' energy fields, I would love to go in this direction with some of you who practice therapeutic touch or other energy work.

7.   In addition to being in the appendixes of this book, the instruments cited above are also available in full text from my web pages and from CINAHL which is a large research database for health researchers available through university libraries on the Web. I would appreciate hearing about any study in which the GCQ (or an adaptation) is being used, and the psychometric properties revealed in your population. I

am also interested in any factor analyses that you perform and will be happy to assist with your articles if you wish (I would request last authorship in cases that warrant more involvement on my part). My e-mail or snail mail address may be used for communicating your use of and findings associated with comfort instruments. (Please initiate contact through e-mail.) In this way, we can build the knowledge base about comfort together.

The Theory of Comfort

Because any study is better with a theoretical base, you can and should use a theory when planning your study. Of course, I would suggest that the Theory of Comfort makes it easy to plan a congruent design that has a good chance of producing significant findings. How to do this, and how Comfort Theory came to be, are topics explored in chapters 4 and 5.

MUSINGS ON COMFORT QUOTE (CHAPTER 3)

> If he paid for each day's comfort with the small change of his illusions, he grew daily to value the comfort more and set less store upon the coin.
> —Edith Wharton (1904), *The Descent of Man*, chapter 1

I chose this quotation because it captures the changeable nature of comfort. The perception of what comfort is and the psychological state in which one perceives comfort determine, in part, the extent of comfort experienced at any given time. Also, I think that this quotation captures a trend where the speaker appraises comfort as being higher on each successive day, given increasing wisdom. Or it could mean that the speaker would give up part of a dream or wish in order to increase comfort. Regardless of the interpretation, we see that comfort is dynamic, an active endeavor, and highly valued.

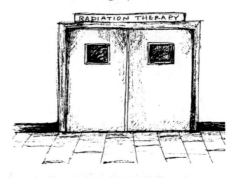

CHAPTER *4*

Philosophical Perspectives

We were camped beside a brook that came down through
marble basins, overflowed down marble cascades, filled
other basins, and overflowed again. The banks, like the
basins and chutes, were clean stone. The sun was out after
two days of rain. We spread out and spent the morning
drying tents, clothes, and sleeping bags. The days before
had been without flaw or jar, even through the rain. . . .
Now we sprawled in swimming suits on the clean marble
while green and white water, veined like marble itself, went
past us. . . . We were utterly at peace, comfortable, indolent,
basking. . . . There we lay, young, healthy, relaxed, without
a care, forgetful of everything except comfort and sun.
—Wallace Stegner (1988), *Crossing to Safety*, p. 199

As I have said before, I often get questions from graduate students
about how to apply Comfort Theory in one of their assignments.
These questions are very helpful because they indicate to me what
clarifications need to be done. Many of these questions are answered on
my Web site in the FAQs section (Kolcaba, K., 1997), reprinted in
Appendix J of this book. But an e-mail inquiry I received recently
requires a more lengthy response. A student wanted to know, "What is
the philosophical perspective of your theory?" This is an excellent question and the answer is an important one to pull together, as there are
pieces of the philosophical perspective in many of my publications.

The first part of this chapter is devoted to answering that question and I discuss three levels of philosophical perspective that were brought to bear on Comfort Theory. The highest level of abstraction, which is the overarching perspective, is that of holism. The next level down is human needs, then comes Murray's Theory of Human Press (1938), and finally three mid-range nursing theorists. From these four perspectives, Comfort Theory emerged. Also included in this discussion is how I define the metaparadigm concepts.

The second part of this chapter is a discussion of how we obtained empirical evidence for the phenomena of holism—the overarching perspective—and what we found. For those readers who don't need to know about these issues right now, jump ahead to chapter 5 and just get into the theory.

HIERARCHY OF PHILOSOPHICAL PERSPECTIVES

Holism

My conceptualization of holism, consistent with my husband's work on the topic (Kolcaba, R., 1997), is person-based. He defined holism as the belief that whole persons consist of a mental/spiritual/emotional life that is intimately connected with their physical bodies. Whole persons are set within complex ecologies, such as social and environmental ecologies, which provide their context for living and experiencing. They perceive the complexities of these ecologies simultaneously and respond instantly, inwardly and/or outwardly.

Persons' bodies comprise their own natural boundaries. They respond mentally, physically, and behaviorally to their immediate surroundings, rather than being one with their surroundings. Whole persons develop knowledge about the world to form a self-concept and an understanding of their place in the scheme of things. They have memories, personalities, ethics, and feelings and are capable of planning for the future.

Assumptions of Person-Based Holism

The assumptions of this conceptualization of holism represent a merger of my previous work (Kolcaba, 1994) with my husband's (Kolcaba, R., 1997). They are as follows:

1. Human beings respond to complex stimuli as wholes.
2. The whole response is greater than what would be expected by examining separate responses to separate stimuli and adding together the effects of those responses.
3. Whole persons do not disappear into ever larger wholes.

Whole-Person Responses

Nurse scientists are beginning to explore the effectiveness of broadly targeted holistic interventions such as progressive muscle relaxation, music and art therapy, massage, guided imagery, and therapeutic touch. These interventions and others are intended to elicit a positive whole-person response and thus would be measured most accurately by a whole-person outcome. A whole-person outcome would measure positive or negative interrelated effects between aspects of that person's response. The instantaneous and comprehensive response would be reported as a total response.

Case Study: Whole-Person Responses

In the following case study, Ted is apprehensive about his upcoming knee surgery. He is afraid of a general anesthetic, pain, blood loss, loss of mobility, and loss of dignity and independence during the procedure and in the postoperative period. All of these separate fears seem rather minor when considered objectively and separately. When Ted experiences them together, while sitting in the waiting room, however, they add up to panic. "This is my body, my surgery, my unknowns. I'm going under the knife!" Ted's whole person response is greater or stronger than if he thought only about immobility one time, blood loss at another time, etc.

Holistic Interventions

Holistic interventions, or complementary interventions, are often used in conjunction with standard medical treatments. When interventions, such as guided imagery, are added to standard treatments, such as surgery or chemotherapy, they can be helpful in decreasing side effects, like bleeding or nausea respectively. These interventions are labeled holistic because they are meant to bring about desirable whole person responses. For this case study, we want to change Ted's holistic panic into a more therapeutic state so that he will fare better in surgery and in the postoperative period.

Nurses and other health care professionals must be able to provide evidence that holistic interventions work by documenting their desired, positive, whole person effects (responses). Holistic outcomes are most congruent with holistic interventions because this type of outcome measures a person's simultaneous responses to his or her surroundings; I call holistic outcomes *immediate*. Comfort is an immediate holistic outcome that is state specific; that is, the patient's state of comfort can change rapidly when circumstances change.

Relationship of Holistic Outcomes to Subsequent Outcomes

In the example of Ted, we could measure his comfort in the waiting room, before anyone stared reassuring him. This would be Ted's baseline comfort, and is called Time 1. Let's say the design of this little study is to have the receptionist give Ted a brief comfort questionnaire to complete along with his other forms. (For an example of questions that might be on a peri-operative comfort questionnaire, see Appendix D. This is a questionnaire that one of my nurse anesthetists created following directions in chapter 3.) Remember that high comfort scores indicate a high degree of comfort.

From the description of his fears, we would expect Ted's total comfort score to be quite low at this initial time point. Then a peri-operative nurse begins working with him, senses his panic, and takes his vital signs (blood pressure, pulse, and respirations are high). He is demonstrating a fight or flight response and would simply just like to get out of there.

Our perceptive nurse talks with Ted about alternatives to general anesthesia and about patient controlled analgesia after surgery. The nurse talks about exercises to strengthen the knee and about the minimal blood loss usually associated with his surgery. The nurse assures Ted that the surgeon will carefully drape him and that the anesthetist will maintain constant supervision over Ted during the entire procedure. Most reassuring, perhaps, is the fact that Ted's nurse will accompany him into the operating room and will stay with him. She fully understands how he feels about his personal dignity and will be his advocate. This is what we would call "usual care" in a research study, although in many cases, patients receive far less than this type of care, or coaching, as it is described in chapter 5.

The nurse can see that Ted is calming down. Ted completes the comfort questionnaire again (Time 2, after coaching) and vital signs are improved. Then the nurse goes the extra mile and begins a guided imagery exercise with Ted. Ted is asked to close his eyes, picture himself in a favorite place, relax his body incrementally, and then imagine the surgery in the most positive ways as suggested by the nurse. "You will feel no pain upon awaking, you will have hardly any bleeding," etc. (In the next chapter I call this type of intervention *comfort food for the soul.*) When Ted completes the guided imagery, he is fully relaxed and confident. He completes a third comfort questionnaire (Time 3), and his vital signs are even better.

The nurse quickly adds up Ted's three comfort scores at each time point (Time 1, Time 2, and Time 3) and notices that his comfort scores steadily improved. "Well, the coaching improved Ted's comfort, but not as much as the guided imagery. And isn't it interesting that his vital signs improved with each time point although there was a bigger change between Time 2 and Time 3 . . . I wonder if increased comfort is related to improved vital signs?" (Statistical analyses can answer this question.) As you will read in the next chapter, the Theory of Comfort posits that the immediate outcome of comfort is related to the subsequent outcome of improved vital signs. Other subsequent outcomes of interest might be postoperative bleeding or pain.

The example of Ted shows why, how, and where we would measure a holistic outcome. The nurse wanted to know if coaching and guided imagery (a holistic intervention) increased Ted's comfort, a holistic outcome. In order to demonstrate that patient comfort is important, not only for the nurse but for the hospital, the nurse also needed to know whether comfort was related to other outcomes that may be considered more significant clinically. There is general agreement that vital signs and blood loss are clinically significant. Other subsequent outcomes might be adherence to rehabilitation regimen, return to previous function, healing of the surgical site, and amount of pain medication. Even further down the road, the nurse could get a copy of Ted's patient satisfaction survey to determine whether interventions to enhance comfort were related to patient satisfaction. It would make sense for hospital administrators to be interested in that relationship. In this way, concepts such as comfort gain importance when they are related to other concepts. Nurses and other members of the health team have rationale for taking the time to enhance patient comfort, in addition to the altruistic reason by which we are usually motivated.

They are also demonstrating that guided imagery improves patient outcomes—a quality improvement issue.

Comfort as a Holistic Outcome

If we look again at Ted's fears, we see that they are interrelated. His fear of a general anesthetic, and of pain, blood loss, immobility, dependence, and indignities during the procedure and in the postoperative period are synergistic, adding together to create panic. These fears can be called comfort needs, and when they are relieved each relieved need is called an aspect of comfort. A comfort questionnaire or visual analog scale measures all of these aspects of comfort at one time. A total comfort score also accounts for the interrelationship of those aspects.

When we say that the whole is greater than the sum of its parts, we mean that one pressing comfort need can detract from total comfort more than might be expected from the nature of the comfort need or other comfort needs that are known. As well, one holistic intervention such as guided imagery can have many interrelated positive effects on enhancing a patient's comfort and achieving desirable subsequent outcomes.

Human Needs

The next hierarchical level in my philosophical perspective is patient needs. It is less broad or abstract than the perspective of holism. Kim (1999) classified nursing theories into three possible categories upon which theorists base their work: (a) human needs, (b) adaptation, and (c) the health/illness continuum. In the first category, human needs, clients are viewed in terms of the state that they are in with respect to what they need or require in order to be sustained or to grow. Such is the second level of orientation for Comfort Theory.

Most scholars agree that humans possess certain organic or "basic needs" that must be satisfied for the sake of physical health (Fortin, 1999). Other academics build on this statement by arguing that people have desires and aspirations extending beyond physiological or somatic needs. Those desires must also be satisfied in order to avoid "dire consequences" (Fortin, 1999). Desires and aspirations such as for social support, staying in one's own home, being understood, being financially secure, and maintaining functional health are entailed in the construct of holistic comfort which embodies physical, psychospiritual, sociocultural, and environmental needs (Kolcaba, 1992b). Because the theory is based on needs of patients, it is a representation of what patients hope to maintain or regain while in the health care system.

Two characteristics of human needs have been identified. First, needs produce a motivational drive that directs human behavior (Fortin, 1999). Patients have implicit and explicit comfort needs that, when met, strengthen and motivate them. Then patients are able to perform better in therapy, heal faster, and adhere more readily to new health regimens. These subsequent results, in turn, enhance comfort (Kolcaba, 1994). Second, needs are a force driven by social and cultural politics (Fortin, 1999). Patients' comfort needs are driven by expectations and cultural norms delineating what is important. Therefore, I believe that patients *expect* health care that is competent, individualized, culturally sensitive, and complete.

Human Press

The efforts of Murray (1938) and colleagues to synthesize major elements of personality theories into a single coherent model led to his Theory of Human Press. Murray called his model "organismic" (an earlier word for holistic) and stated, "Since the parts of a person cannot be dissected physically from each other, and since they act together, ideally they should all be estimated simultaneously" (Murray, 1938, p. 46). Murray defined needs as drives induced by obstructing forces that prompted activities designed to satisfy the drives (1938). If needs are addressed successfully by appropriate interventions, the immediate outcomes are perceived by the person as being, "on the whole," relatively positive. The third philosophical level is Human Press.

According to Murray, a stimulus situation consists of alpha press and beta press. Alpha press is the sum of negative (obstructing) forces, positive (facilitating) forces, and interacting forces. Beta press is the person's *perception* of the total effect of the forces in alpha press. For health care, obstructing forces are the total negative stimuli arising from the health care episode, including side effects of illness or treatments; noxious or threatening environmental and social experiences; and emotional sensations such as fear, anxiety, powerlessness, or aloneness. The facilitating forces are interventions designed to address needs that remained after the person's own reserves were depleted by obstructing forces (Kolcaba, 1994).

As stated above, beta press is the person's perception of the total effect of the phenomena in the stimulus situation. The events in the situation are interpreted as a temporal gestalt of stimuli which could be either threatening or reassuring. Beta press includes the appraisal of how well the needs that arise from the obstructing alpha forces are met by facilitating forces in the stimulus situation. When the outcome is positive, self-evaluations (by patients) accumulate and provide the expectation that other situations will end positively. This expectation is called a unitary trend, and it can be positive or negative based on past experiences (Kolcaba, 1994). Using a process called substruction, I made a preliminary diagram of Murray's concepts which then provided a conceptual framework upon which to "hang" concepts related to comfort and health. That diagram provided the basis for Comfort Theory as described and illustrated further in chapter 5.

Nursing Theorists

Comfort Theory originated in and for nursing. Only recently have I thought about the theory being appropriate for members working together on a health care team, which I hope will be the prevailing model of care in the 21st century (see chapter 9). The fourth philosophical level, therefore, is nursing.

Three nurse theorists contributed directly to the understanding of the Three Types of Comfort that evolved. Orlando (1961/1990) discussed the extant comfort needs of patients and the nurse's ability to assess and address those needs. When the needs were met, patients would experience *relief*. The nurse assessed the patient's physical and mental comfort, before and after a comfort measure was delivered. The nurse accomplished this through an effective nurse-patient relationship. This process consisted of careful observation and utilization of the principles that Orlando developed in her interaction theory.

Henderson (1978) described 10 basic physiological and psychological functions of human beings that had to be addressed by nurses in order to maintain homeostasis of patients. They were respiration; nutrition; elimination; body mechanics including transportation and prevention of pressure sores; rest and sleep; keeping clean and well groomed including dressing and undressing and protection of integument; controlling the environment for optimal atmospheric conditions including sanitation, esthetics, and protection from infection and other dangers; communication including human relations, learning, health goals, and guidance; work and play; and worship. If homeostasis in these categories was maintained, persons would be in the comfort state of *ease* (my derivation from Henderson).

Paterson (Paterson & Zderad, 1976/1988) stated that comfort is a construct that communicated the nature or experience of nursing. She believed that comfort was an umbrella under which all other nursing terms could be sheltered, such as growth, health, freedom, and openness. (As noted in chapter 2, Gropper [1992] later echoed the idea that health is comfort.) Because Paterson was a psychiatric nurse, she defined comfort from a mental perspective rather than from a physical one, although she acknowledged that mental and physical comfort were interrelated. Her definition of comfort was

> a state valued by a nurse as an aim in which a person is free to be and become, controlling and planning his own destiny, in accordance with his potential at a particular time in a particular situation. (Paterson & Zderad, 1976/1988, p. 101)

Paterson called the freedom to be and become, *transcendence.*

Other theorists who discussed comfort less directly were Peplau (1952), Watson (1979), and Roy and Roberts (1981). Peplau mentioned comfort in conjunction with other human needs such as food, rest, sleep, companionship, and understanding (1952). Roy and Roberts stated that the nurse employed traditional comfort measures to achieve comfort or relieve discomforts in the physiological mode (1981). Watson called comfort a variable that affected external or internal environments and that comforting activities could be supportive, protective, or corrective (1979). All of these usages provided different views about what comfort was, but comfort was not defined in the theories or nursing diagnoses, except for Paterson and Zderad's existential characterization of the term (above) (1976/1988).

Metaparadigm Concepts

Fawcett (1984) defines a metaparadigm as a statement or group of statements identifying the relevant phenomena of a given discipline. These statements include discipline-specific central concepts and themes. The purpose of a metaparadigm is to establish boundaries and describe the topics for study in that discipline. Some theorists challenge Fawcett's definition and others wonder if she has correctly identified nursing's metaparadigm. Regardless of these disagreements, Fawcett's work has withstood the test of time.

Fawcett stated that there are four metaparadigm concepts for the discipline of nursing: person, environment, health, and nursing (1984).

More recently, the concept "person" has been utilized as client, patient, family, community, region, or nation—where ever nurses practice. The term "nursing" can mean the discipline (noun) or what nursing does (the verb). Fawcett did not define the concepts, but rather stated that it was the responsibility of individual theorists to define them, according to their perspective and assumptions. Therefore, I have included my definitions of each concept below, congruent with the perspectives previously described.

Often, when students discover Comfort Theory, and find its extensive Web site (K. Kolcaba, 1997) including a link to my e-mail address, they ask me how I define the metaparadigm concepts. This is another good question. Here follows, from the FAQs section of The Comfort Line (Appendix I), my own definitions of the metaparadigm concepts:

> *Nursing:* the intentional assessment of comfort needs of patients, families, or communities; design of comfort measures to address comfort needs, including re-assessment of comfort level after implementation of comfort measures, compared to a previous baseline
> *Patient:* an individual, family, or community in need of health care, including primary, tertiary, or preventive care
> *Environment:* aspects of patient/family/community surroundings that affect comfort and can be manipulated to enhance comfort
> *Health:* optimum function of a patient/family/community facilitated by enhanced comfort

These definitions are congruent with Comfort Theory and evolve as the theory evolves.

EMPIRICAL EVIDENCE FOR THE NATURE OF HOLISTIC COMFORT

We saw, with the example of Ted earlier in this chapter, that the goal of holistic interventions is for many desirable changes to be experienced simultaneously by recipients. These changes might include increased relaxation, positive thinking, images of success, and feelings of well-being and contentment. Whole-person changes like these may be temporary but are consistent with the complexity of human experience. To measure such complex outcomes with separate instruments is time and energy consuming and creates artificial partitioning of whole-person responses.

The outcome of comfort is a holistic state that captures many of the simultaneous and interrelated aspects of positive human experience. In numerous clinical research settings, enhanced comfort is a desirable and meaningful outcome. In the examples of infertility (Schoener & Krysa, 1996), immobilization after cardiac catheterization (Hogan-Miller, Rustad, Sendelbach, & Golderberg, 1995; Keeling, Knight, Taylor, & Nordt, 1994), chronic obstructive pulmonary disease, and radiation therapy for early-stage breast cancer (Kolcaba & Fox, 1999), multiple mental and physical discomforts are experienced although physical pain is minimal. Patients in these situations hope to have their complex comfort needs addressed. Nurses and others respond by providing holistic interventions that complement the medical regimen. Assessments of comfort before and after these interventions can demonstrate whether the interventions are effective. Instruments to assess comfort also provide data that give us insight into the nature of holistic responses (Kolcaba & Steiner, 2000).

In chapter 3, the proposition was explored that comfort could increase over time given an effective and consistently applied intervention. The opportunity for this exploration was my dissertation and the setting was radiation therapy (RT). Women with early-stage breast cancer participated in the study and, in most cases, they already had a lumpectomy. Participants were randomized into two groups. One group listened to an audiotape of guided imagery every day for the duration of RT and for 3 weeks afterwards, while the other group received usual care. Comfort was measured with two types of instruments at three time points: Time 1, before RT began; Time 2, in the middle of RT, and Time 3, 3 weeks after RT was complete.

We discovered that, indeed, comfort was higher in the women receiving guided imagery compared to women receiving usual care. In addition, we used data from that breast cancer study to test two theoretical propositions about the nature of holistic comfort. The additional propositions that we tested in secondary analysis were these:

1. Does the outcome of comfort have more *state* characteristics than *trait* characteristics?
2. Is the whole (Total Comfort) greater than the sum of its parts (Relief, Ease, and Transcendence added together)?

To review the methods of this study in more detail, please go back to chapter 3.

Review of the Instruments

1. *Radiation Therapy Comfort Questionnaire (RTCQ)*. This instrument was adapted from the original General Comfort Questionnaire (GCQ). The RTCQ was designed to measure whole person responses of women going through RT for early-stage breast cancer. The 26 items in the final RTCQ were distributed across the content domain of comfort and there were positive and negative items to reduce response bias (see Appendix B). The response set was changed from four responses in the GCQ to six responses in the RTCQ to increase sensitivity (Jenkins & Taber, 1977; Oaster, 1989; Rasmussen, 1989). Anchors for the Likert-type scale ranged from strongly agree to strongly disagree as on the GCQ. Scores on the RTCQ met assumptions for parametric testing and demonstrated a Cronbach's alpha of .76 (Kolcaba & Fox, 1999; Kolcaba & Steiner, 2000).

2. *Visual Analog Scales (VASs) for Comfort.* The VASs were developed primarily for the reason of establishing preliminary concurrent validity with the RTCQ, as there were no established measures of holistic comfort to use for that purpose. There were other advantages, however, with using VASs. First, it was difficult to capture all aspects of any concept in a given questionnaire and an abstract concept such as comfort, with all of its meanings and usages, is especially difficult to capture. Therefore, we thought that VASs might better represent the personal uniqueness and richness of the concept for the study participants (Youngblut & Casper, 1993). Second, there was a very wide range of possible responses on the VASs because the woman's placement of her mark on the VASs is measured in millimeters. Because most VASs are 10 cms. (100 mms.) in length, there are 100 different possible scores. Because of the range of possible scores, VASs can be quite sensitive.

Three vertical VASs were labeled Relief, Ease, and Transcendence to signify factors derived from the earlier factor analysis of the GCQ (Kolcaba, 1992b). When scores from these three scales were added together (total mms. for the three scales), a measure for the parts of comfort was derived and labeled Summed Comfort scales. An additional VAS was created for Total Comfort (TC). Stems for the VASs went like this: TC, "I feel as comfortable as possible right now;" Relief, "I have many discomforts right now;" Ease, "I am feeling at ease right now;" and

Transcendence, "I am feeling motivated, determined, and strengthened right now."

The length from the low end of the lines to the patient's mark was measured in mms. Relief was reverse coded because it was worded negatively. Data from all VASs were skewed to the left, indicating that participants responded consistently with higher comfort scores. Means and standard deviations for each VAS were computed at Times 1, 2, and 3. The standard deviation (SD) for TC over three time points averaged 1.58, whereas the SD for the Summed Comfort scales over three time points averaged 5.19.

Answering the Research Questions

The first research question was this:

1. Does the outcome of comfort have more *state* characteristics than *trait* characteristics? To determine the extent of state versus trait characteristics in this population, Heise's method (as cited in Knapp, Kimble, & Dunbar, 1998) was used with data from the RTCQ. Only data from the control group were included to remove the effects of the intervention. Trait stability of comfort was calculated by comparing test-retest correlations at three time points according to specific formulas for each interval in the longitudinal data (Knapp et al., 1998). Reliability coefficients with numbers closer to 1.00 demonstrated higher trait stability. Reliability coefficients were as follows: between Time 1 and Time 2, .63; between Time 1 and Time 3, .40; and between Time 2 and Time 3, .53. Thus, trait stability was variable between time points and not particularly dominant (Kolcaba & Steiner, 2000).

We also obtained intraclass correlation coefficients that measured within-subject time differences (Shrout & Fleiss, 1979). Intraclass correlations for control group data were obtained over the three time points. Results were TC, .38; Relief, .45; Ease, .44; and Transcendence, .59. Thus, results across measurement points were interpreted as having a relatively low degree of repeatability with Transcendence having the highest degree. (It may be that the characteristic of being able to transcend stressful situations is more of a character trait while needs for Relief and Ease are more state-specific.) Time seemed to have a moderate effect on comfort scores as recorded on the VASs. These findings supported the earlier results with the RTCQ, that is that comfort generally has a higher proportion of state characteristics (Kolcaba & Steiner, 2000).

The second research question was this:

2. Is the whole (TC) greater than the sum of its parts (Relief, Ease, and Transcendence added together)? We thought that we could approach this question by testing the hypothesis that the VAS scores for TC (the whole) in the treatment and control groups would demonstrate significantly greater comfort than Summed Comfort scales (sum of the parts) at each time point. To do this, the means for TC (in mms.) was compared to the means for Relief (after reverse coding), plus Ease plus Transcendence. The following proportion was created:

$$\frac{\text{Relief plus Ease plus Transcendence}}{300 \text{ mm.}} = \frac{X}{100 \text{ mm.}}$$

The expected score if the whole was the same as the sum of its parts was called X or expected. Then, X was compared to what the women actually marked on the TC line. If TC was significantly greater than X, the holistic tenet that total comfort is greater than the sum of its parts (Relief, Ease, Transcendence) could be accepted. (Mathematically, the proportion pictured above is the same as dividing relief plus ease plus transcendence by 3 and comparing the result with TC (Kolcaba & Steiner, 2000).

Data from the VASs for Relief, Ease, and Transcendence (Summed Comfort scales) were compared to data from the VAS for TC using the Wilcoxon signed rank test. Differences between the paired samples of the Summed Comfort scales and the TC scale were highly significant ($p = .00$) at all three time points. Our hypothesis was supported. Thus, the whole (total comfort) was significantly greater than the sum of its theoretic parts (relief plus ease plus transcendence) and the synergy between parts in relation to a complex whole was demonstrated (Kolcaba & Steiner, 2000).

DISCUSSION ABOUT QUANTIFYING HOLISTIC COMFORT

Although participation in this study was offered to all women who met the inclusion criteria, the women who consented were alert and vigorous. Their ages ranged from 37 to 81 years and there were 7 minority and 46 Caucasian women. They all found the VASs fast and easy to use, compared to the 26-item RTCQ. The broad nature of the stem for TC ("I am as comfortable as possible right now"), however, failed to be sensitive to differences in holistic comfort between women and between groups. The narrow average standard deviation across three time points (1.58) was indicative that the women all answered within a very narrow range on the 100 mm. line. Although comfort means different things to different people, in the absence of pain other components of comfort seem to flatten the differences between individual responses. There was much more variability in each of the Summed Comfort scales, indicating that when meaning is narrowed a bit, women had different responses.

For future explorations of comfort, I would suggest collecting more triangulated data. This strategy combines the strengths of quantitative and qualitative findings about the comfort of specific populations. In the breast cancer study, women kept diaries for when they listened to their guided imagery (GI) audiotapes and any other comments they wanted to include. These diaries were a rich source of qualitative data that I discussed extensively in my dissertation, and to a lesser extent in Kolcaba and Fox, 1999. For example, the finding that state anxiety was positively related to comfort at baseline was not expected. In talking to the women, though, I found that those who were highly anxious reached out urgently to friends and family for self-preservation. That is, they asked for and received help in various forms of social support. At baseline then, before any interventions or bonding with RT staff or the nurse researcher, these anxious women were actually more comfortable because of the positive effects of the social support that they sought. This phenomena speaks to the adaptive properties of anxiety, and also to the interrelatedness of comfort components. Without the qualitative data, the relationship between anxiety and comfort would have been difficult to understand.

Comparing data from VASs and traditionally formatted comfort questionnaires will continue to be important. Each type of comfort instrument offers different information and has different strengths. The traditional format is more reliable for quantitative data analysis. VASs are easy to use, however, and the idea of a patient reporting his or her own comfort on a real or imaginary scale from 1 (low) to 10 (high comfort) is appealing for clinical use. VASs enable nurses to begin conversations with patients about their comfort, asking them to identify distracters from comfort should they report a low comfort score.

MUSINGS ON COMFORT QUOTE (CHAPTER 4)

> We were camped beside a brook that came down through
> marble basins, overflowed down marble cascades, filled
> other basins, and overflowed again. The banks, like the
> basins and chutes, were clean stone. The sun was out after
> two days of rain. We spread out and spent the morning
> drying tents, clothes, and sleeping bags. The days before
> had been without flaw or jar, even through the rain. . . .
> Now we sprawled in swimming suits on the clean marble
> while green and white water, veined like marble itself, went
> past us. . . . We were utterly at peace, comfortable, indolent,
> basking. . . . There we lay, young, healthy, relaxed, without
> a care, forgetful of everything except comfort and sun.
> —Wallace Stegner (1988), *Crossing to Safety,* p. 199

This quote speaks to the holistic nature of comfort. The possibility of
physical pain is not an issue, and yet comfort is real, palpable, and
experienced with full awareness that yes, *this* is comfort. We get the
sense that these friends are being soothed and strengthened by the
comfort they feel and that their sensations are, indeed, transcendent.

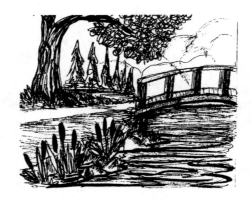

Theoretical Explorations

> It must never be lost sight of what observation is for. It is not for the sake of piling up miscellaneous information or curious facts, but for the sake of saving life and increasing health and comfort.
>
> —Florence Nightingale (1859, p. 70)

In chapters 1, 2, and 3, I described how the definition of comfort and a map of its content domain, called the taxonomic structure (TS), were developed. From the TS, the General Comfort Questionnaire (GCQ) was developed and subjected to an instrumentation study as a pre-dissertation exercise. In chapter 4, I discussed the philosophical underpinnings of Comfort Theory. In chapter 5, we will explore how comfort relates to other concepts, such as health, as Nightingale implied in the above quote. When we explore these relationships, we are really "theorizing." How this theorizing led to the Theory of Comfort is the topic of this chapter.

DISSERTATION CONTINUED

At the time of the instrumentation study (chapter 3), Dr. Roberts and I were surprised that the GCQ had a Cronbach's alpha of .88, because brand new instruments usually don't perform that well. We also were delighted that the factor analysis supported the TS of comfort by finding three factors or subscales of comfort: Relief, Ease, and Transcendence. In retrospect, I believe both occurred because the instrument was derived from a well researched TS. In addition, our heterogenous sample provided some evidence of the wide applicability of the concept across patient populations, ages, and cultures. Whether on a medical-surgical unit or at home, persons from diverse backgrounds enjoyed answering questions about their own comfort. They related to each question because each was meaningful to their daily experiences. I was confident that the attributes of comfort had been well represented by the TS.

I barely had breathed my sighs of relief at having finished the instrumentation study and the galleys for the article about the GCQ (Kolcaba, 1992b), when Dr. Roberts surprised me with the "suggestion" of doing an experimental study for my dissertation. As described in detail in chapter 3, it took me about a year to choose a population with acute comfort needs that would be amenable to a holistic intervention (women with early-stage breast cancer going through radiation therapy), a holistic intervention that I could target to the population's specific comfort needs (guided imagery), a way to deliver the intervention consistently and with sufficient repetition to effect change (audiotape and tape player), a way to measure comfort in my specific population (Radiation Therapy Comfort Questionnaire [adapted from the GCQ] and four visual analog scales), a study design that could demonstrate a trend for increasing comfort given an effective intervention, and a method of data analysis that could detect differences over time between the treatment and control group (Repeated Measures Multivariate Analysis of Covariates). These were major, difficult, and time consuming decisions and every possible choice had ripple effects on other choices to be made.

Once those decisions were made, however, I needed a theoretical framework—a requirement for every nursing dissertation out of Case Western Reserve University (CWRU). Prior to my dissertation, I had an outcome, comfort, that I could measure—that's all. I next chose the components for my future study that would be congruent with comfort. I still didn't have a theory, though. To say that my process was backward would be accurate and the fact that I led with the caboose has had its difficulties throughout my career, but that's the way it was.

The philosophical perspectives discussed in chapter 4 were foundational for the Theory of Comfort. The process of theory development was built on that foundation in three stages: induction, deduction, and retroduction. This chapter contains details about the first two stages. The third stage is discussed in chapter 9, because it occurred much later in the process. That's one of the fun things about theory development—the theory evolves and accommodates changes in reality.

DEVELOPING A MID-RANGE THEORY OF COMFORT (KOLCABA, 1994)

What Is a Mid-Range (MR) Theory?

An MR theory is not a broad or grand theory which is abstract, complicated, and removed from practice and research. MR theories are meant to be easily grasped and applied. Compared with grand theories, MR theories contain fewer concepts and relationships, are adaptable to a wide range of practice and experience, can be built from many sources, and are concrete enough to be tested (Whall, 1996). For these reasons, MR theories are particularly cogent as the science of health care addresses challenges of the 21st century.

When thinking about a theory of comfort, I felt that it would be at the mid-range level because that was the level of my early dementia framework (Kolcaba, 1992a) as described in chapter 1. As I reviewed the concepts in that framework, I was thinking inductively.

Induction

Induction occurs when generalizations are built from a number of specific observed instances (Bishop, 1998). In the late 1980s, I was head nurse on an Alzheimer's unit. I was familiar with some of the concepts used to describe the practice of dementia care: facilitative environment, excess disabilities, optimum function. When I drew relationships between them, however, I recognized that these three terms did not fully describe my practice. There was an important piece that was missing and I thought about what we were doing on the unit to prevent excess disabilities in order for patients to function optimally. The activities entailed in optimum function made our residents feel good about themselves if it was the "right" activity at the "right" time (a few times a day). What were they doing in the mean time? What behaviors did we, the staff, hope they would exhibit that indicated an *absence* of excess disabilities?

Answering these questions required close observation and analysis and eventually brought the term comfort to the forefront of my thinking. When I introduced comfort to the original diagram it was because this word conveyed, for me, the desired state for patients to be in when they were not engaging in optimum function. This type of thinking was the first step toward identifying comfort as an important concept for health care. As stated previously, the concept analysis that followed resulted in three types of comfort (Relief, Ease, and Transcendence) derived from three nursing theorists respectively: Orlando (1961/1990), Henderson (1978), and Paterson (Paterson & Zderad, 1976/1988). See chapter 4 for a complete description of the contributions that these theorists' work made to my understanding of comfort.

The next step was to relate comfort to other nursing concepts. This relational kind of thinking is deductive.

Deduction

Deduction is a form of logical reasoning in which specific conclusions are inferred from more general premises or principles; it proceeds from the general to the specific (Bishop, 1998). I didn't have a general set of premises, though, upon which to hang the three types of comfort. I needed an abstract and general conceptual framework that could be congruent with the lesser concept of comfort and which contained a manageable number of highly abstract concepts. These concepts would provide the context for patient comfort in health care. No grand theory of nursing could accommodate the diverse work of the three nursing theorists who provided the foundation for Relief, Ease, and Transcendence. Therefore, I had to look elsewhere for common ground that could unify the three types of comfort.

The Work of Henry Murray

An organizing framework for comfort had to meet the following criteria. Because the TS of comfort was based on needs (chapter 4), the organizing framework had to link (a) needs arising from health care situations of (b) whole persons for whom health care professionals could intervene. The effectiveness of (c) the interventions had to (d) be perceived by those persons (patients) and (e) be related to subsequent outcomes (Kolcaba, 1994).

Where to find such a conceptual framework (CF)? For my dissertation, I couldn't just create a CF out of whole cloth, as our program required that we add to existing knowledge. So I started looking at dissertations in our library, to see what former students had used. I came across Margaret England's dissertation and saw that she used Henry Murray's theory to formulate her own model about caregiving. (You might recall from chapter 1 that Margaret had already influenced me in the development of the taxonomic structure.) Margaret did not diagram Murray's theory, however, nor did Murray himself. Fortunately, I had learned about substruction from Dr. Eileen Morrison and I found that diagramming was a very useful exercise for designing a study, at least for me. After I diagrammed Murray's major concepts, they appeared to be a great fit with comfort and with my dissertation population, women with early-stage breast cancer. (Preliminary discussion about Murray's theory is in chapter 4.) It was highly abstract, inclusive, and holistic. (It also didn't hurt that Dr. Roberts, my dissertation chair at the time, was Margaret's dissertation chair, too.)

Because Murray's theory was about human press, it was applicable to patients who experienced multiple stimuli in stressful health care situations. A new diagnosis of breast cancer certainly fit the description of health care as being stressful and with multiple stimuli. In the model of human press, a stimulus situation was that part of the total environment to which people attended and reacted during a given episode in their life. Human development, whether positive or negative, was determined by the accumulated impressions about one's success or failure that were formulated during encounters with the situation. For the level of mid-range theory, I defined a stimulus situation as any health care situation.

For health care, I defined alpha press as the sum of negative (obstructing) forces, positive (facilitating) forces, and interacting forces. Beta press is defined as the patient's perception of how well the nursing interventions (facilitating forces) meet comfort needs arising from the health care situation (obstructing forces) for which the patient requires assistance to satisfy. Perceptions of enhanced comfort lead to the reinforcement of habits and goals that are successful in reducing negative tensions (Kolcaba, 1994). (The possibility of a trend for increasing comfort given an effective and consistent intervention is entailed in Murray's work.)

Patterns of successful habits and goals led to an orienting thema that provided direction for future action (Murray, 1938). A desirable thema that nursing and other health care providers seek to promote is a health thema that I defined as the patient's general orientation to health seeking behaviors (HSBs). The concept of HSBs was first explicated by our former nursing dean at CWRU, Rozella Schlotfeldt (1975). I proposed that a reciprocal relationship existed between HSBs and comfort because HSBs could also enhance comfort (an insight from one of my undergraduate clinical students who was using the theory with her patients). Schlotfeldt conceptualized HSBs as internal, external, and a peaceful death. Internal behaviors occurred at the cellular or organ level, such as healing or immune function. External behaviors were observable, such as self-care, function, and rehabilitation. My definition of a peaceful death was one in which conflicts are resolved, symptoms are well managed, and acceptance by the patient and family members allows for the patient to "let go" quietly and with dignity (Kolcaba & Fisher, 1996). The relationships between these concepts are diagrammed in Figure 5.1.

Murray's concepts are found in lines 1, 2, and 3 of Figure 5.1. From these concepts, I continued the process of substruction, diagramming the most abstract concepts at the top under which are placed concepts that are increasingly concrete. Referring to Figure 5.1, *Line 1* consists of concepts that are very abstract and sometimes difficult to define; *Line 2* consists of concepts that are less abstract and may be subdivided to make them easier to define; *Line 3* consists of concepts that are more concrete than in line 2, but still generalized to any discipline and setting; *Line 4* consists of concepts that are specific to nursing and health care but are general in terms of clinical setting. (The clustering of the first three concepts in lines 4 and 5 designate that these measures are analyzed together in a multivariate analysis of variance. There is more about this method of holistic data analysis in chapter 7.) Note that line 4 represents Comfort Theory; it is no longer Murray's Theory of Human Press. The diagram shows that there are three types of HSBs. In chapter 9, I will demonstrate how to continue substructing for outcomes research within specific clinical settings.

The deductive process for constructing this theory consisted of substructing from Murray's abstract theoretical concepts to more specific health care concepts in a logical manner. Because comfort is perceived by patients it was logically substructed under Murray's concept of "perception." Murray's concept of "health thema" then led naturally to Scholtfeldt's concept of HSBs.

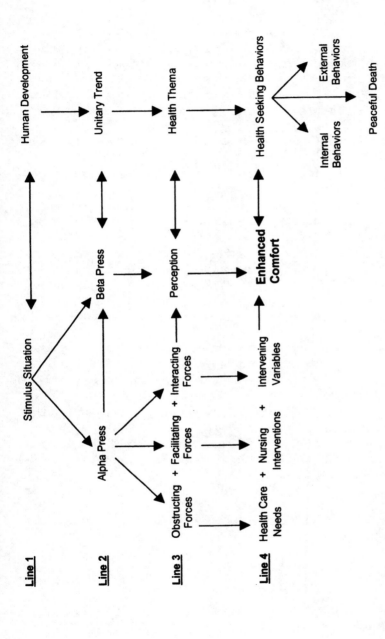

FIGURE 5.1 Comfort Theory substructed from the Theory of Human Press.
Used with permission of Blackwell Publishers. From Kolcaba, K. (1994). A theory of holistic comfort for nursing. *Journal of Advanced Nursing, 19,* 1178–1184.

"Obstructing forces" were substructed as health care needs (for holistic comfort), "facilitating forces" were interventions or comfort measures, and "interacting forces" were intervening variables. Line 4 shows a positive relationship between interventions and enhanced comfort. This proposed relationship is the first and altruistic part of the Theory of Comfort. The theory is *normative* (what nurses and other team members *should* do) and *descriptive* (what team members *do* do, if they subscribe to this theory). Propositions for the first part of the theory are:

1. Nurses and other team members identify patients' comfort needs that have not been met by existing support systems.
2. Nurses and other team members design interventions to address those needs.
3. Intervening variables are taken into account in designing the interventions and determining whether they have probability for success.
4. If the intervention is appropriate, and delivered in a caring manner, the patient experiences the immediate outcome of enhanced comfort. *Comfort Care* entails (a) an appropriate intervention, (b) delivered in a caring (comforting) manner, and (c) with the intentional goal of enhanced comfort.

The last column of the diagram addresses the question, why comfort? For nursing and health care, "unitary trend" was substructed to health thema, which was further substructed to HSBs. Some examples of HSBs are improved functional status, better response (or effort) in therapy, faster healing, or a peaceful death. Thus, the theory states that patients who are comfortable are more likely to engage in HSBs, which determine in large part their level of wellness or peacefulness of death. The idea that patients will do better if comforted successfully provides rationale for nurses and others to engage in Comfort Care. Propositions for the second part of the theory are

5. Patients and nurses agree upon desirable and realistic HSBs.
6. If enhanced comfort is achieved, patients are strengthened to engage in HSBs. Engagement in HSBs further enhances comfort.

Miscellaneous Comments

At this point in the process of theory development, I had a two-part nursing theory that I could and did use for my dissertation study. The first part theorized that nurses developed interventions to enhance comfort and the second part was relating comfort to subsequent HSBs. The diagram proved to be a valuable aid as it directed me to explicate the needs of women with early-stage breast cancer, think about intervening variables that might have an impact on the outcome (such as age, marital and financial status, number and ages of children, etc.), design an intervention congruent with the outcome, and make sure the outcome covered the content domain of comfort, which is the immediate desired outcome. I thought briefly about possible subsequent outcomes and whether I wanted to add them to my study. I decided, however, to focus my energies on my main research interest, which was to demonstrate with statistical significance that comfort increases over time in a group that receives an effective and consistent nursing intervention. (I also needed to focus on graduating!) In deciding to limit my inquiry, I think I set the stage for other nurse researchers to do the same; that is, test one part of the theory at a time, at least in the beginning of one's research program. In fact, I think it is a practical strength of Comfort Theory. As I have since learned, comfort studies in any given population can dominate one's research program very quickly.

I soon realized that Murray's abstract framework combined with my nursing concepts constituted a new theory of nursing. I showed the diagram (Figure 5.1) to Dr. Roberts and she approved it for my dissertation. The theory was also presented at the Midwest Nursing Research Conference to get professional and diverse feedback, and I subsequently incorporated many of those insights. Then the article was sent to *Journal of Advanced Nursing*, which had published the concept analysis paper earlier. They accepted it quickly and the Theory of Comfort was in the literature (Kolcaba, 1994).

Dr. Youngblut was aware that the Theory of Comfort had been published. She said an interesting thing that I still pass on to my students. She said, "Concepts are not interesting in and of themselves. It is placing them in context with other concepts that makes them come alive. That's what you did when you developed your theory. You needed to do that to make comfort relevant." Ah, the power of theory . . . I am constantly reminded of its importance.

Another comment about Comfort Theory that I remember was received during my dissertation defense, about 3 years later. Dr. Shirely Moore, a member of my committee, asked if the work of Henry Murray should be utilized more in nursing, because it had been so useful to me (and others). My reply was, "I don't think it's necessary to promote

Murray's theory for nursing, rather I see Comfort Theory as being a mid-range theory that stands alone. Murray provided a useful framework, but I think nurses will be interested only in lines 4 and 5 of the diagram." Now, as I am asked to apply the theory to new settings, I use only lines 4 and 5 because I believe they exemplify the breadth and scope of a mid-range theory. Murray's work was also limited as far as advancing the theory for the 21st century. I needed to go beyond him in a process called retroduction. This third stage of theory development will be described in chapter 9.

Referring now to Figure 5.2 on the next page, line 5 is a more concrete level of the theory because it depicts concepts that are definable in a narrow and useful way for research. I call this level a micro- or practice level theory. Micro-level comfort theories serve as conceptual frameworks for practice, education, and research and are publishable as such. Line 5 is the operational level, or how each concept in the theory is measured or implemented. The naming of the instruments for measurement of each concept is the most concrete level in any substruction and is usually placed at the bottom of the diagram.

COMFORT CARE AND COMFORT MEASURES

While preparing presentations for a perianesthesia nursing conference and an end-of-life seminar, I took a fresh look at the idea of comfort care (Kolcaba & Wilson, 2002). I concluded that Comfort Care entails at least three types of comfort measures that I hope all nurses and other team members will keep in mind, whether or not they subscribe to this theory:

1.   *Technical comfort measures* are those interventions designed to maintain homeostasis and manage pain, such as the monitoring of vital signs and blood chemistries. It also includes administration of pain medications. These comfort measures are designed to (a) help the patient maintain or regain physiologic function and comfort, and (b) prevent complications.

2.   *Coaching* is a comfort measure designed to relieve anxiety, provide reassurance and information, instill hope, listen, and help plan realistically for recovery, integration, or death in a culturally sensitive way. For coaching to be effective, it must be timed well to capture a patient's readiness to accept new thoughts (Benner, 1984).

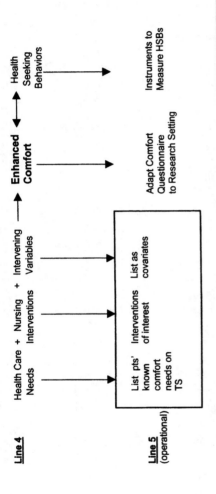

Line 4

Health Care + Nursing + Intervening → **Enhanced** ↔ Health
Needs   Interventions   Variables   **Comfort**   Seeking
                                                            Behaviors

Line 5
(operational)

| List pts' known comfort needs on TS | Interventions of interest | List as covariates |

Adapt Comfort Questionnaire to Research Setting

Instruments to Measure HSBs

Propositions in Original Theory of Comfort

1. Nurses identify patients' comfort needs that have not been met by existing support systems.
2. Nurses design interventions to address those needs.
3. Intervening variables are taken into account in designing the interventions and determining whether the have probability for success.
4. If the intervention is effective, and delivered in a caring manner, the immediate outcome of enhanced comfort is attained. Comfort Care entails these three components.
5. Patients and nurses agree upon desirable and realistic HSBs.
6. If enhanced comfort is achieved, patients are strengthened to further engage in HSBs, which further enhances comfort.

FIGURE 5.2 Mid-Range Theory of Comfort.

Used with permission of Blackwell Publishers. From Kolcaba, K. (1994). A theory of holistic comfort for nursing. *Journal of Advanced Nursing, 19*, 1178–1184.

3.   *Comfort Food for the Soul* are those comfort measures that are unexpected by today's patient, but so very welcome because they entail old-fashioned and basic nursing care. Like comfort food that you eat, these comfort measures make patients feel strengthened in an intangible, personalized sort of way. Comfort food interventions target Transcendence through presencing and memorable connections between nurse and recipient, who might be one patient, a patient and/or family, or a group. Suggestions for comfort food for patients include massage, environmental adaptations to enhance peace and tranquility, guided imagery, music therapy, reminiscence, and hand-holding. These are the interventions that fortify patients for difficult tasks. Today's nurse often doesn't have time to provide comfort food for the soul but these types of comfort measures are facilitated by a commitment to Comfort Care by the institution (see chapter 9). I believe this is how nurses really want to practice, and if they are given the opportunity to do so, promotes greater nurse creativity and satisfaction as well as high patient satisfaction.

In order to enhance comfort, the nurse must deliver the appropriate intervention in a caring manner. Sometimes when the appropriate intervention is delivered in an intentional and comforting manner, however, comfort may still not be enhanced sufficiently. When this happens, the nurse looks at the intervening variables for reasons that comfort care is not working. Such variables as abusive homes, lack of financial resources, devastating diagnoses, or cognitive impairment may render ineffective the most appropriate interventions and comforting actions.

As stated earlier, the construct of Comfort Care includes intervention, comforting actions, and the goal of enhanced comfort. It is intentional. This is much different than the usual connotation of comfort care as an advance directive, thought of as a last resort in many institutions. Our Comfort Care is proactive, energized, intentional, and longed for by patients and families in all settings! An evaluation of Comfort Theory, done by a professor of nursing and colleague, is in Appendix J.

MUSINGS ON COMFORT QUOTE (CHAPTER 5)

> It must never be lost sight of what observation is for. It is not for the sake of piling up miscellaneous information or curious facts, but for the sake of saving life and increasing health and comfort.
>
> —Florence Nightingale (1859, p. 70)

In this quote, Nightingale implied that life, comfort, and health were different but related and equally important goals of health care. She believed that nurses were responsible for these patient outcomes. Nurses take calculated, informed actions to promote these outcomes based on their observations of patients. Theorizing about the relationships between concepts such as health and comfort helps to clarify why and how nurses and other team members do what they do.

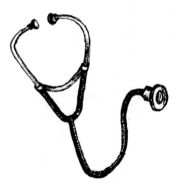

Attributes of Comfort[*]

> I define comfort . . . as that warm, safe feeling you get from
> lying in bed watching the rain fall, knowing you don't have
> to go out of the house if you don't want to. Comfort is also
> that vital, connected feeling you get when you talk openly
> with your partner or a close friend. Comfort is a place to
> fortify yourself for upcoming or ongoing struggles and for
> the challenge of inner work. . . . Above all, I define . . . com-
> fort as self-acceptance.
> —Jennifer Louden (1992), *The Woman's Comfort Book*, p. 2

Have you noticed that comfort is a very "in" word these days? It
seems to appear everywhere—in advertising, secular writing,
and politics. Perhaps this appeal to comfort is a collective cultural response to our feelings of personal alienation in a very stressful
world. Technology has a depersonalizing effect. Additionally, in society,
government, and health care, capitalistic values and insecurities make
us feel vulnerable and insignificant. In the absence of satisfactions in
the social realm, we seek to create feelings of comfort by softening our
immediate surroundings. The above quotation, in fact, comes from "a
self-nurturing guide for restoring balance in your life" and implies
that self-comfort can be an antidote to our fast-paced, uncertain lives
(Louden, 1992). (Fortunately, the author promotes only constructive

---

[*]This chapter written in collaboration with Dr. Raymond Kolcaba.

and healthy self-comforting activities.) The quote also speaks to the need that humans have for comfort, the fact that comfort is positive and strengthening, and that it is an active endeavor.

The increasing cultural desire for comfort has a few drawbacks from my point of view (although in general, I'm happy about the trendiness of comfort). One drawback is that the concept could come to mean almost anything. Actually, Louden is citing a few examples of comfort rather than defining it—a strategy many use when the concept they want to define is very abstract. Louden could have given us any of a boundless group of other examples, or instances, of comfort. Even so, the process of multiplying examples leaves open what comfort is. Just what makes these examples instances of comfort? Just about anything could be said to be comforting in some circumstances under some conditions.

When a term comes to mean almost anything, it loses its ability to designate something specific. Comfort could be applied to so many situations, things, and relations among things, that it loses its capacity as a descriptor. If everything is a part or cause of comfort then nothing is special. Comfort would be ever present and inescapable. What we are concerned with here is this: When comfort is advertised in connection with hospitals or home care, what in particular does comfort specify?

This chapter is intended to remedy the lack of clarity in the use of comfort by showing how the *technical* definition of comfort for health care specifies attributes and boundaries of the concept. For constructing research studies or clinical ladder projects, you will want to have a clear understanding of what you are measuring or trying to improve. Also, for student assignments in theory or research classes, this chapter will be helpful, not only for the extended analysis of comfort but as a guide for analyzing other concepts as well.

I hope this entire book speaks to the continued value of patient comfort as a nursing goal and a goal for health care in general. From nursing's roots and for nursing's future, may we be convinced that comfort is important to patients! As most illness-related situations are so stressful, comfort is that much more essential for recipients of health care than, say, for baseball fans in a ballpark.

THE NATURE OF CONCEPT ANALYSIS

How then can we approach the concept of comfort? In general, concepts arise from two main sources: as new ideas in science and from our cultural and linguistic heritage. The concept of DNA is an example of a new idea in science because it was unknown until recently. The concept of DNA started as a technical idea in biochemistry. Concepts such as comfort and health, however, are part of our cultural heritage. The concepts of comfort and health started as ideas in our ordinary language and are applied to our ordinary experience.

If we want to define scientific concepts like DNA, we would go to its context of use. We would go directly to theories in chemistry and biology in which DNA plays a role. The boundaries of the concept of DNA are of interest to a research scientist. Some of these boundaries are the causal links to other processes of reproduction, some of which are still unknown. Empirical research will further reveal boundaries of the concept of DNA.

If we want to define cultural concepts like comfort, we would begin by tracing its linguistic history. The Oxford English dictionary provided a semantic basis for the origin of the concept of comfort and was utilized heavily in our original concept analysis. Then we examined contemporary dictionary definitions to determine what nuances were dropped, which were retained or built upon, and which meanings are first, second, third, in common understanding. We also needed to explore the many usages of the concept, both ordinary and disciplinary, technical and informal, past and present. These three methods are discussed in our concept analysis article (Kolcaba & Kolcaba, 1991).

Analysis involves examining the parts of something. We break down a reality in order to understand how its parts are interrelated. In the case of a concept, we examine the parts of the concept and try to grasp how it is organized. Exploration of the boundaries of a concept take us *beyond* analysis. This is an important exercise because delimiting boundaries of concepts helps us understand where one concept leaves off and a different concept begins. Boundaries determine the meaning of a concept.

When we examine boundaries, we go beyond looking at parts of a concept to looking at its relations with a wide variety of *other* concepts. So, in addition to concept analysis, we could do conceptual explication, conceptual exemplification, and conceptual comparisons. Walker and Avant, in their well-known text *Strategies for Theory Construction in Nursing* (1988, 1995), utilize an encompassing notion of concept examination (which they call "analysis") that focuses on these other activities. An interesting exercise would be to analyze their concept of concept analysis!

Suppose a concept analysis *did* include delimiting the boundaries of a concept. Then, a subtle shift in reference has occurred: the *object* of the analysis has changed from the target concept to the target concept as part of a group of concepts. The object of analysis has come to include the relationships among concepts in the group. Therefore, in order to keep the object of analysis constant, that is, to avoid the shift in reference we prefer to say that when we go beyond a concept, we are *explicating* the relations between that concept and others. These relations reveal boundaries of the target concept. Explorations of the relationships among concepts presuppose an understanding of the concepts that are related. If we understand those concepts and the target concept, we can grasp some of the boundaries between them.

In doing a conceptual *explication*, then, we may need first to become clear about the target concept. For research purposes, a concept like DNA is, now, perhaps clear enough to most, although in the early years, research was needed to discover its properties. For lay purposes, the concept of DNA needs no further analyses. What about a concept like comfort? The extent and type of analysis depends on the goal of the analysis. For our first concept analysis of comfort (Kolcaba & Kolcaba, 1991), we wanted to define the term in a technical way for health care research and practice. From that technical definition, the problem was tackled of how to measure changes in patient comfort as the result of nursing care.

It is timely for us to build on our concept analysis of comfort (Kolcaba & Kolcaba, 1991) by explicating some of its boundaries. Walker and Avant present some useful strategies for this type of inquiry. Many students have asked me, via Email, to assist them with their classroom assignments that are modeled after Walker and Avant's work. In this chapter, with some commentary to qualify our methods, we will perform their exercises that involve: (A) choosing the concept, (B) determining the aims or purposes of analysis, (C) identifying uses of the concept, (D) discussing defining attributes of comfort, (E) constructing cases (model, borderline, related, contrary, invented, and illegitimate), (F) identifying antecedents and consequences, and (G) talking about empirical referents (Walker & Avant, 1995). First, though, let's clarify what a concept is.

WHAT IS A CONCEPT?

An important point to remember in any concept analysis is the difference between a concept and examples of that concept in the world.

Car is a concept. This red sedan is an example of the concept car, as is that white convertible or this yellow "beetle." These three examples of cars look very different from each other but they share the *attributes* that make them cars. Among other things, they all have tires, a certain size chassis, a horn, starter, transmission, etc. The concept of *car* entails these attributes and refers to examples of cars in the world, the red sedan, white convertible, or yellow "beetle."

We all think we understand the boundaries of the concept of car. But think about the debate surrounding sports utility vehicles (SUVs). Most of them are actually built on small truck chassis which are bigger and heavier than car chassis. Congress declared that trucks could have lower emission standards so they could move goods more economically across our vast country—but owners of SUVs aren't performing this economic function. Therefore, are SUVs really trucks? Is function an attribute? SUVs share one defining attribute of trucks, a small truck chassis, and they are larger and heavier than is indicated by our usual concept of car. The boundaries of this concept, car, have blurry edges! These blurry edges have caused problems with resource management and the economy.

The distinctions among concepts, attributes, and examples are important when doing a concept analysis because concepts specify attributes, refer to examples, and have boundaries. All of this reveals that a concept is an abstract notion with attributes of some concepts being attributes of other concepts. A concept is useful when its attributes are clear, its definition sets boundaries, and it specifies a *unique combination* of attributes that no other concept has.

Remember, the concept specifies its attributes and attributes designate examples in the world. The examples in the world are not the concept. (Walker and Avant speak otherwise by saying that concepts occur in the world.) To continue with our analogy, the *concept* of car doesn't honk. The red sedan in the world honks. The attributes specify the boundaries of the concept. Many people, such as Louden in our opening quote, confuse examples of a concept with the concept itself. So understanding the attributes, rather than the examples, is essential for understanding the concept. To include all examples of the concept would then make the concept undefinable.

Interestingly, Walker and Avant (1988, 1995) do not ask for a definition of the concept of interest at the end of their exercises. We believe this is a weakness in their methods. Our feeling is that a successful analysis of a concept should result in, at least, a provisional or working definition of the concept. Because we have already published a technical definition of comfort for the discipline of nursing, we repeat it here so you can respond to it as we go through Walker and Avant's methods for concept analysis. Let's determine if this definition of holistic comfort has clear and useable boundaries, and if examples in the world are representative of its attributes as contained in the technical definition. The technical definition of comfort is *the immediate experience of being strengthened by having needs for relief, ease, and transcendence met in four contexts (physical, psychospiritual, social, and environmental).*

CONCEPT ANALYSIS ASSIGNMENT PER WALKER AND AVANT (1988, 1995)

A. Select a Concept

We have selected Comfort for further analysis.

B. Aims or Purposes of Analysis

This is an important step because the aims or purposes of an analysis decide its nature and extent. Walker and Avant are correct in indicating that pragmatics drive analysis. They leave out, however, that an analysis could potentially omit a number of their steps.

Our purpose is to confirm our earlier definition and examine the possibility of additional boundaries of the concept. We wish to (a) determine whether the TS is a sufficient explication of the defining attributes of comfort in parts A–D, (b) explore boundaries of comfort in parts E and F, and (c) discuss measurement issues in part G.

C. Identify All Uses of the Concept

This third step is feasible only when the number of uses is relatively small. Walker and Avant state that the analyzer must identify *all* the usages, both ordinary and scientific, first because considering broad usage "is likely to yield richer meanings" (Walker & Avant, 1988, p. 39). Then a decision can be made, if necessary, to narrow the usages to those pertinent for science (we would be more specific and say health care science here). As noted above, comfort has become very popular in contemporary culture, but many of the examples do, in fact, support the rich meanings entailed in my definition above. So here is a sampling of examples of comfort from contemporary U.S. sources, followed by brief observations about their meanings.

1. "I ask you to seek a common good beyond your comfort." (President George W. Bush, quoted in *The Plain Dealer*, 2001, p. 1). This example of comfort is the pleasing human state from which we can begin to accomplish greater goals and from which we sometimes don't want to move. Here, comfort does not seem to be a motivating force, but rather one that can delay action and limit orientation to others' needs if one so chooses. So I think the element of choice is raised: we can choose to stay in our comfort zone, or we can use our comfort zones as a source of strengthening for necessary tasks.

2. A journal entitled *Caregivers' Comfort: A tool that would inspire and motivate primary caregivers to be at their best, regardless of the day-to-day circumstances. . . . It is a healing tool* (Downing, 2000). This example of comfort is in the title of a diary that the author constructed to motivate and inspire caregivers to perform difficult and long-standing tasks. The intent of the book is to heal or relieve emotional pain, exhaustion, fear, and frustration associated with caregiving.

3. "I began my day watching as she drew her last breath, then comforted her family in mourning her death," from "A Day in the Life of a Nurse" by Tim Halloway (2001, p. 54). Here, comfort is used as a verb and refers to a process. The example is a nurse doing his job and it implies a prior need (grief) to which the nurse responds in a sensitive and caring way. The nurse's intention is to comfort the family.

4. *Pain Management: Comfort with Caring* is a brochure from the MetroHealth System (1998). This example is an advertising pamphlet that promises relief from pain which is achieved in a caring way. Patient comfort is the focus. The tag line implies that pain is complex and can be decreased with psychological interventions (caring).

5. "Seeing the familiar sights of home after a long journey, I feel comfort and contentment stirring within me. . . . Yet I know wherever I am, God's presence is with me" (*The Daily Word*, 2001, p. 45). This example of comfort is a sense of ease, facilitated by one's familiar environment. Physical discomfort associated with sitting in a car for a long time is transcended by arriving home. There is a spiritual implication that God is present in the car and at home.

6. "It is our intention to make our home a safe, comfortable, family-oriented facility so every trip to Jacobs Field is most enjoyable," says Dennis Lehman, Indians Executive Vice President of Business of the

Cleveland Indians in *Game Face* (2001), the summer program for the Cleveland Indians home games. This form of comfort is an adjective and the example of comfort is the experience at the ballpark. It implies pleasing furniture, atmosphere, food, and facilities. The example doesn't seem to refer to interactions with personnel, but rather the environment at Jacob's Field facilitates pleasing interactions with family members.

7.   "Comfort and presence as you contribute to the larger health care community are expectations of today's nurse executive. . . . Comfort comes through involvement as information is brought to and taken away from these gatherings" (Ferguson, 1989, p. 298). This example of comfort is the sharing of valuable information in social interactions. No secret agendas! The nurse executive is expected to bring such comfort to others and receive it through others.

8.   "When the first driver was ready to turn off in another direction, he sent word to another truck driver to watch over us! It was very comforting for us as we traveled" (Krueger, 2001, 10-E). This is from a Dear Abby column. Here comfort is an adverb and implies an end state. Even though the author did not know or see any of the truckers, she felt comforted by their words of encouragement over CB radios. The example of comfort is the presence of the truckers which strengthened her and her two daughters for their trip and gave them courage as they traveled unknown highways. The unknown causes discomfort.

9.   "The amount of relief and comfort experienced by [the] sick after the skin has been carefully washed and dried is one of the commonest observations made at a sick bed" (Nightingale, 1859, p. 53). Florence Nightingale highlights the importance of the bath as an example of enhanced patient comfort. The carefully administered bath promotes ease and relieves unnamed, but implicitly severe, discomforts.

10.   "Oh, the comfort—the inexpressible comfort of feeling safe with a person" (Craik, 1969). This example of comfort, from a poem called *Friendship*, is the safe haven a trusted friendship provides.

11.   "We must educate so that pain and symptoms are controlled and the patient is comfortable" (Laurie, 2001). This phrase was found in a Letter to the Editor in *The Plain Dealer*. This example is similar to item 6 because comfortable is an adjective, but here it refers to a patient instead of a place. Here the author is talking about the patient being in a state of comfort, which clearly consists of more than pain and symptom management.

12.   "Comfort is the key to looking good in summer—that, and allowing yourself a chance to chill out." In this advertisement for sum-

mer clothes in *Family Circle* (August 7, 2001, p. 73), a young, curvaceous model is wearing a sexy dress, and she is standing barefoot on a beach with the ocean in the background. This example of comfort is the feeling of self-confidence that comes when we know we look great, our clothes fit perfectly, and we are enjoying a favorite place.

13.   "Even though I walk through the darkest valley, I fear no evil; for you are with me; your rod and your staff—they comfort me." This favorite Old Testament verse (Psalm 23:4) demonstrates an example of the spiritual nature of comfort. In this beautiful metaphor, we (sheep) are comforted by God (the shepherd) and his presence gives us strength, courage, and a sense of safety.

14.   Let us not forget the comfort quote at the beginning of this chapter by Jennifer Louden:

> I define comfort . . . as that warm, safe feeling you get from lying in bed watching the rain fall, knowing you don't have to go out of the house if you don't want to. Comfort is also that vital, connected feeling you get when you talk openly with your partner or a close friend. Comfort is a place to fortify yourself for upcoming or ongoing struggles and for the challenge of inner work. . . . Above all, I define . . . comfort as self-acceptance.

Here the examples of comfort are environmental, psychological, and social. In these examples, comfort fortifies Louden for upcoming struggles. She also states that comfort is satisfaction and contentment with oneself.

D. Determine Defining Attributes

Defining attributes are characteristics of comfort that appear over and over again in the examples (Walker & Avant, 1988, p. 39). The above 14 examples of comfort in the world are fairly representative of the different usages of the concept, in nursing and ordinary language. We see that comfort is used frequently, and it has several meanings. We could continue to find other examples, but they probably would duplicate usages that represent the attributes of comfort relevant for nursing. Walker and Avant tell us we can decide to choose more than one meaning for analysis which I believe, for comfort, is necessary because the concept is so rich. As we go we will attempt to validate the technical definition of comfort, as delimited by the taxonomic structure.

First of all, three types of comfort are evident among the 14 examples. For example, *Ease* is in statements 1, 5, and 6; *Transcendence* in statement 2; *Relief* of pain in statements 4 and 9 (note that both of these are from health care). Note that comfort comes from different places: It is *physical* in statements 4, 9, and 11; *psychological* in statements 2, 3, 9, and 12; *spiritual* in statement 13 (there are many references to spiritual comfort in the Bible); *social* in statements 7, 8, 10, and 13; and *environmental* in statements 5 and 13. Can all of these usages of comfort be organized on the TS? Let's find out.

We'll put them on a grid with the three types of comfort across the top and the different places from which comfort arises down the left side to form a grid. The cells that result are the attributes of comfort. Let's see if we can plot the examples of comfort from our 14 statements on the grid (Table 6.1). No fair! We all know that the defining attributes of comfort were tailored to fit the TS that was developed many years ago. In truth, though, the TS seemed a convenient, natural way to depict the complexity of the concept then and we think it is now. There are many attributes of comfort to account for, and most of them are essential for fulfilling the mission of nursing. Some attributes nurses intuitively address and others might have been forgotten but all are worthy of resurrection and implementation. *All* of these components are important to patients.

As we did this exercise, we could literally hear objections or questions arise. (It's the first time we have extended the concept analysis in this way.) To answer your concerns, we have written some possible questions below, with our responses. If you have more questions or objections about the process or outcome of this extension of our concept analysis, please Email *kolcaba@uakron.edu*. Your feedback helps this work evolve and remain relevant.

TABLE 6.1   Examples of Comfort Plotted on Taxonomic Structure

	Relief	Ease	Transcendence
Physical	4, 9, 11	5, 6, 9, 11, 14	2, 9
Psychological	7, 8, 9, 11, 12	1, 5, 6, 7, 8, 9, 11, 12, 14	2, 13, 14, 9
Spiritual	13	1, 5, 13, 14	5, 13
Social	4, 7, 8, 9, 13	1, 7, 8, 9, 13, 14	8, 9, 13, 14
Environmental	5, 10, 13	5, 6, 10, 14	2, 5, 13, 14

Questions From the Audience About This Part of the Analysis

1. *What about the fact that many of the examples can be fit in to several places?*
Comfort is holistic—the examples of comfort affect many attributes of comfort all at one time. Boundaries between the attributes are permeable. The cells in the grid are not mutually exclusive, but rather they have an "and/or" quality. Remember also, not every usage of the term is clear and precise—the above writers were not using our technical definition!

2. *Some examples appear only a few times and others are all over the grid.*
To some extent, this is a function of the senses of the attributes. Some are more universal in scope than others. For example, how environmental comfort affects me is different than how it affects you.

3. *Some qualities of comfort that reappear frequently in the statements aren't accounted for by the TS. For example, comfort often seems to be associated with safety, and it's desirable, temporal, healing, and very personal.*
Some of these qualities (desirable, temporal) are built into the definition. Not every use of the term results in a correct usage, though. We would argue, for example, that comfort is not the same as self-acceptance, which is contrary to what Louden stated previously in example 14. Other qualities that we saw in the examples actually provide rationale for comfort (healing, safety) and were built into the theory later as health-seeking behaviors.

4. *This grid (in chapter 6) looks different than the one in chapter 1 and that you published (Kolcaba, 1991). This one has one more row.*

5. *How did you separate psychological and spiritual comfort?*
We'll answer these two together. Because examples of psychological and spiritual comfort *are* so difficult to separate, they were eventually combined into one context of experience called *psychospiritual* (see chapter 1). So, instead of 15 cells in the TS as in this chapter, the final TS has 12 cells. What was even more difficult was to develop *separate* questionnaire items for psychological and spiritual, an issue that is coming up in this concept analysis. Therefore, it became evident that psychological and spiritual attributes of comfort had so much overlap that it was impractical to try to separate them.

6. *Do your examples contain all of the attributes of comfort that are relevant for a technical nursing definition?*
We think so. Can you find an example of comfort that is relevant for nursing that isn't entailed in the TS? Or more to the point, can you find a nursing example that isn't entailed in the TS? If so, please let us know. We are very willing to make necessary adjustments.

7. *So, what are the defining attributes of comfort?*

Each of the 12 cells of the final TS is a defining attribute. Thus, there are 12 defining attributes of comfort: physical relief, physical ease, physical transcendence, et cetera.

8. *Did you organize examples or meanings of comfort on the grid? Aren't they the same thing?*

We organized *examples* of comfort on the grid for this chapter. We wanted to see whether the TS worked for this purpose. These were examples of usages of the concept in the world. Trips to Jacobs Field (statement 6) is an example of a positive baseball park experience. The bath (statement 9) is an example of patient relief from unnamed discomforts. Each example has its implied meaning, but the meaning is a culturally derived abstraction while the examples are real.

9. *What about the different forms of comfort in the examples (comforted, comfortable, comforting)?*

The different forms of comfort represent ways in which we organize our language. These forms are examples of patient comfort only if, in the context of any sentence in which the forms appear, the term comfort refers to outcomes or end states. (This is the distinction between process and product as described in chapter 2.) The TS defines the boundaries of the *outcome* of comfort. But statement 3 describes the process of comforting by nurses and therefore, because it is not an example of an outcome, the term comforting is not on the TS. We don't know if the family was truly comforted (because no one asked them), but we know the nurse tried to comfort in a caring way and this, in itself, is often comforting. Here, comforted is not an outcome, it is a process. On the other hand, the statement "I was comforted by the nurse" is about an outcome that was realized.

10. *Aren't you being arbitrary in your placement of the examples of comfort on the grid (Table 6.1)? I would place them somewhat differently.*

Personal experience with comfort helps guide our judgments and personal experience varies among persons. An appeal to that experience should result in a good reason for a judgment. Then it is not arbitrary.

11. *How can you tell when someone is demonstrating the attributes of transcendence?*

Transcendence is such an important goal for nurses, but how can we tell if we are successful? Many people, in fact, don't want to move from ease to transcendence, as George W. Bush implied in statement 1. Transcendence means that one has risen above difficult work or circumstances but oftentimes, he or she would just not be in a position to put out that kind of effort! When the going gets tough, though, and when we have no choice, as when chemotherapy or painful postsurgical physical therapy are necessary, transcendence might be the only way to get through the nightmare. How can the nurse tell if he or she has achieved this laudable goal for nursing? Well, the patient keeps going. If you're lucky you might get a thank you, but usually you just know. Helping a patient achieve transcendence can be the most rewarding and challenging function of nursing.

E. Developing Cases

The reason for developing cases is to discover whether they reveal anything new about the boundaries of the concept. We found the exercise to be useful and creative, but somewhat problematic for the following reasons. First, how are students to know what kind of case to develop if they do not have a definition of the concept in place? We rely on our understanding of the concept through knowing about its attributes. In other words, cases presuppose the meaning of the term. For example, when developing a contrary case, students without a prior definition might ask, "Contrary to what?"

Second, thinking of cases also presupposes understanding the attributes of borderline concepts. Other concepts may need to be defined and analyzed before proceeding with the development of model cases. Because we had our technical definition, however, we were able to proceed with the assignment. Below are our candidates for cases:

Model Case

A model case is a pure instance of the concept, a paradigmatic example (Walker & Avant, 1988, p. 40). The following vignette contains excerpts from a favorite article of mine that appeared in *Cleveland Nursing Weekly* a few years ago. It was written by Gerald Humphreys and reprinted from the November 1989 issue of the *American Journal of Nursing*. I believe it embodies a model case for holistic comfort as experienced by a real patient. (Italics were added by me to highlight use of the concept in question.)

Dear Nurse,
You are responsible for my recovery, I hope you will remember that
... You were key to my overcoming the odds, of beating the coronary

artery disease that all but ended my life. . . . It was you who gave me the will to live. . . . You gave me the enthusiasm I needed to accept and to adapt.

As I see it, you excelled in the things that, simple as they are, physicians cannot always understand. In ICU . . . you always had a smile for me. You squeezed by hand and told me I was doing well. *You comforted me.* I will never forget how suddenly buoyant I felt when you took my vital signs and gave me a good report . . . I felt you were proud of me and I did not want to disappoint you. . . .

In the bustle of the cath lab, you stand out in my memory as an eye of calm in the midst of a storm. You draped me and washed me with antiseptic, all the while telling me exactly what to expect and how to handle it. . . . You prepped me for surgery, encouraging me all the way. . . . Even in the numbing atmosphere of the postoperative ICU, when a person who cannot talk or swallow can easily reach the edge of panic, you were there. You hovered over me, softly *comforting,* yet all the while measuring and monitoring. . . .

Even now, I choke back tears as I try to tell you what your words and gestures meant to me . . . you were my contact with the reality of wellness. And you never failed to help. . . .

This model case contains examples of Relief, Ease, and Transcendence that occur physically, psychospiritually, socially, and environmentally. Comfort was the holistic outcome and the patient used the words, "You comforted me." We know that the comforting actions worked.

Borderline Case

Borderline cases are those examples that contain some of the critical attributes of the concept being examined but not all of them (Walker & Avant, 1988, p. 40). In thinking about a borderline case, I was reminded of an encounter I saw when I was a staff nurse about 10 years ago. I was taking care of my patient in a double room and the patient in the other bed had an IV. His nurse came in to change the bag, and she had an efficient way about her that I admired. We were well staffed that day, but she still maintained her speedy efficiency. She came in, told her patient she was going to change his IV, and did it in the blink of an eye. She had no trouble resetting the pump, of course, smiling and making the technological part of her job look easy. The patient wasn't terribly sick, in fact he was pleasant and quite glad to see her. After about two minutes, however, she left as quickly as she had done everything else, just as the patient was literally opening his mouth to ask her a question. His question never had a chance. This efficient nurse provided some attributes of comfort when demonstrating her technical competence and friendliness, and when she left her patient's environment was neat. She failed, though, to provide psychospiritual support or social comfort through listening, responding, and caring.

Related Case

Related cases are examples of concepts that are related to the concept being studied but that do not contain the critical attributes (Walker & Avant, 1988, p. 41). *Safety* is my candidate for a related case. Like comfort, safety has other word forms such as safely, is safe, and safe. It is listed as a noun in the dictionary, as in "Patient safety is important," but it is used also as an intransitive verb, as in "My patient is safe." Patient safety is an important value for nurses, so much so that RNs campaign for patient safety as a main reason to improve staffing. Physical safety implies freedom from injuries, including falls, medication errors, undiagnosed or misdiagnosed complications, nosocomial infections, et cetera. Environmental safety implies well maintained equipment and furniture, nonslippery floors, cleanliness, lack of noxious fumes, etc. Social safety implies that our patients are under our protection from psychotic or criminal behavior, family disruption, false information, and negligent or nasty personnel. In addition to these attributes, patients can experience relief (a specific danger removed) or ease, where safety is maintained.

A comfortable environment is not the same thing as a safe environment, though, and one can be safe but not comfortable. Also, a critical attribute of comfort, transcendence, is missing in safety. Thus, safety is a very different concept from comfort. The two concepts are on the same level of abstraction, they both are important nursing values, and they both are complex and comprehensive, but there is a warm, fuzzy, and motivating quality to comfort that we don't find in safety. Also, comfort is more self-aware; we know whether we are comfortable, but we don't always know whether we are safe.

Invented Case

An invented case is constructed using ideas outside our experience (Walker & Avant, 1988, p. 42). This might seem an unusual way to think about comfort, but here is an example. A beautiful beach house was built overlooking the dunes and ocean in South Carolina. It was designed, I think, to resemble an unfurled banner. From the beach, the house had five sections that tapered from left to right, which was the direction of the prevailing winds. Each section was successively smaller and each was topped with a bright green roof. We beachgoers called it the House With Five Green Roofs and, like a banner, it served as my family's landmark when we strayed from our beach chairs, towels, and other family members.

During the day the House was dignified and solid, but since it was designed as a banner, it wasn't content to be so still and stiff. So, during every full moon, the house got its wish to be transformed into a real banner and it fluttered gaily in the breeze, under the moonlight. It was free to be and become all that it was meant to be—a lovely banner, a landmark full of motion, life, and welcome. The House transcended its solid state through the intervention of the full moon. Only when it fulfilled its destiny as a banner did the House feel truly comfortable about itself.

An editorial comment: Having never applied comfort in an imaginary way, I found this to be a poetic exercise, and I enjoyed it. At first I thought I had not learned much from this case, but in reflection I believe that when the House came alive in my imagination, the *essence* of comfort was expressed—the whole gestalt that occurs when the House achieved its fullest potential. Our House existed in a state of dignity but not in a state of transcendence. Through the magic of the full moon, the House became all it was meant to be. In doing this exercise, I came to believe that the attributes of transcendence make comfort truly special and unique as a desired goal for nursing. What do you think?

Contrary Case

Suffering is a concept that is decidedly *not* comfort and I think that if comfort is on one end of a continuum, suffering is at the other end. Suffering is the opposite of comfort and nurses must try to alleviate suffering wherever they can. Consider this: A man with end-stage renal failure has no family advocate or advance directives to help facilitate a peaceful death. He slips in and out of consciousness as his organs fail one by one. His renal failure is being treated aggressively in a high-tech procedure called Continuous Veno-Venous Hemofiltration. Statistically, his chances for recovery are extremely slim, but he has no means to remove himself from aggressive care. His bedsores are painful, and the invasive lines frequently become infected or clogged. When he is conscious he does not speak coherently. The environment is confusing, noisy, always lit. This man suffers constantly from his physical problems and from his internal desperation.

We can learn something new about comfort when we consider its opposite, suffering. First, it is unethical to allow patients to suffer thusly because we are disregarding their rights of autonomy and we are disregarding our obligation for beneficence by allowing suffering. Moreover, suffering is an antecedent to wishes for suicide or euthanasia.

Consider another possible contrary case: A husband is madly in love with "another woman." His wife is sickly and spends most of her time in bed. She manipulates her husband to take care of her and rather enjoys her success as an attention-getter. The husband wants out, but his wife is "too sick" for him to request a divorce. One night this desperate man says to his bedridden wife, "Here darling. Let me fluff your pillow and make you *comfortable.*" She smiles weakly and gazes up at her husband with helplessness and trust. He removes the pillow from behind her damp hair, fluffs it, and places it firmly over her face, smothering her to death.

In writing this second and different type of contrary case, the husband just plain lies. Is this a contrary case? The husband is using the term "comfortable" incorrectly and is actually seeking his own comfort, albeit unethically and immorally. In constructing this case, I realized that in providing true comfort, intent makes a big difference. Clearly, the intent of the husband was not to provide comfort. I think this is true in nursing as well, because when nurses implement their interventions, if there is no intent to comfort along the way, the interventions often do not comfort, even when they are technically appropriate.

Illegitimate Case

An illegitimate case is defined by Walker and Avant as an example of the term used improperly or out of context. It is difficult to distinguish this case from the contrary case, and perhaps that is why Walker and Avant say that this last type of case is not always included in classroom assignments or articles. As an example for the nursing concept of coping, they give "coping saw," and the semantics of the term seem to be the issue. A "comfort station," as a euphemism for an outhouse, may be one type of illegitimate case. A second type of illegitimate case might be a sadomasochist who is *comforted* by receiving painful whippings. Here, this bizarre form of comfort is the manifestation of an illness or abnormal need. In addition, this example is one of process (that which comforts), while the product of the recipient's comfort might be real, but nevertheless, unhealthy.

Analysis of Model Cases

In the scenarios above, we did not discover any additional defining attributes. We already knew there were areas of overlap because, by the very nature of holistic comfort, the attributes are interconnected. We did not discover areas of contradiction between the attributes. Rather the cells in the TS work together to convey the gestalt of patient comfort. Was this extension of our previous concept analysis (Kolcaba & Kolcaba, 1991) useful? I believe it was because it helped me to explicate the essence of comfort. Specifically, the importance of intentionality and transcendence were emphasized through the exercise.

Developing model cases and explicating antecedents and consequences also assists in discovering the essence of the concept, boundaries of the concept, and theoretical relationships with other concepts. Other questions still remain, however: Were new boundaries of comfort discovered? Why not take logically opposite concepts and pinpoint their essential differences, such as the differences between suffering and comfort? Or look at a family of similar concepts and pinpoint their differences, for example differences between consolation, support, and comfort?

The result of the assignment, for me, was to confirm in a new and different way (a) the adequacy of the TS of comfort for specifying the attributes of comfort, (b) the accuracy of the technical definition of comfort in delimiting boundaries, and (c) the usefulness of Comfort Theory to describe relationships between comfort and other nursing concepts.

F. Identify Antecedents and Consequences

Walker and Avant (1988) state that something cannot be an antecedent and an attribute at the same time. This is helpful to clarify, and caused me to think about the antecedents and consequences of comfort and how they relate to the Theory of Comfort. I discovered that both antecedents and consequences were embedded in the theory, but not stated as such. Perhaps, identification and consistency between antecedents/consequences is a good test of the logic of a theory. In any case, because Comfort Theory has been around for a while, it was easier for me to explicate antecedents and consequences than it would be for concepts that have not been previously defined or set in a theory.

Antecedents

To reiterate, the 12 attributes of comfort, as designated by the TS, comprise the state of Total Comfort. In order to enhance Total Comfort, nurses intervene for comfort needs that have not been met by the patient or his/her natural support system, using the TS as a guide. Patients have needs for Relief, Ease, and Transcendence and these can occur physically, psychospiritually, socioculturally, or environmentally. The needs exist whether or not the nurse cares or is aware, so the assessment of comfort needs in four contexts is critical to getting the process started. Assessment (intuitive or formalistic) precedes intervention; the length of time between assessment and intervention depends on the nurse's assignment, motivation, or skills to act on the assessment. Thus, *interventions to enhance holistic comfort* are the antecedents closest to comfort. It is important to remember that the goal of Comfort Care is to enhance comfort above the baseline assessment; it is probably not realistic to think that nurses can provide Total Comfort in a stressful health care setting.

Consequences

The consequence of enhanced patient comfort is the patient's engagement in health seeking behaviors (HSBs), as stated in the Theory of Comfort (Kolcaba, 1994). HSBs can be internal, external, or a peaceful death (Scholtfeldt, 1975). Internal HSBs are not visible from the outside, but many indicators are available through lab work. Examples are immune parameters (such as the number of T-cells or natural killer cells), homeostatic mechanisms such as oxygen saturation or blood pressure, peristalsis, and cardiac output. External HSBs are visible behaviors such as ambulation, functional status, successful discharge, or adherence to a medical regimen. A peaceful death is one in which conflicts are resolved, symptoms are well managed, and acceptance by the patient and family members allows for the patient to "let go" quietly (Kolcaba & Fisher, 1996). The extent of comfort is positively and directly correlated to the extent of patients' engagement in HSBs and this relationship has been tested empirically.

G. Specify Empirical Referents

Walker and Avant (1995) state that empirical referents are classes or categories of actual phenomena that by their existence or presence demonstrate the occurrence of the concept itself (p. 46). An empirical referent for the concept is the same as an operational definition of the concept and both terms refer to a research instrument. Thus, the empirical referent that I use to measure general comfort is the General Comfort Questionnaire. Other researchers, including myself, have different instruments for measuring comfort in various settings, as shown in Table 3.1.

We can also say that each attribute of the concept has its own empirical referent; that is, each question on a questionnaire is designed to refer to an attribute of the concept. In order to make sure all the defining attributes of a given concept are measured, a map of the content domain (all attributes) is recommended (Lynn, 1986). The TS is a type of content map and it facilitates inclusion of relevant empirical referents for each attribute. So the TS directs us to generate items from each of the 12 cells. An example of physical relief is, "I am able to walk." An example of environmental transcendence is, "This view inspires me." The General Comfort Questionnaire has 48 empirical referents, approximately 4 for each of the 12 defining attributes. In keeping with general guidelines for instrument development, there are even numbers of positive and negative items for each attribute (or cell on the grid), which reduce response bias.

MUSINGS ON COMFORT QUOTE (CHAPTER 6)

> I define comfort . . . as that warm, safe feeling you get from lying in bed watching the rain fall, knowing you don't have to go out of the house if you don't want to. Comfort is also that vital, connected feeling you get when you talk openly with your partner or a close friend. Comfort is a place to

> fortify yourself for upcoming or ongoing struggles and for
> the challenge of inner work. . . . Above all, I define . . . com-
> fort as self-acceptance.
>
> —Jennifer Louden (1992, p. 2)

While the above quote presents wonderful examples of comfort, they
are not definitions of comfort. For clarity in thought, writing, and
speaking, it is important to distinguish between examples of a concept
and attributes of a concept. Examples are instances or uses of the
concept in real life. Attributes are those qualities that, taken together,
specify the unique characteristics and help set boundaries of a concept.
From a discovery of the defining attributes of a concept, we can generate
conceptual and operational definitions of a concept that are essential
for testing theoretical relationships between the primary concept and
other concepts.

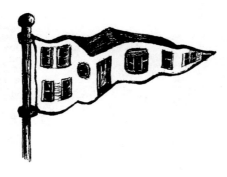

The Experiments

They knew luxury, they knew beggary, but they never knew *comfort.*

—Samuel Johnson, 1750
(letter about making a living through writing)

Chapter 7 begins with a discussion of conceptual and operational definitions, both of which are essential for experimental studies. Then four comfort studies that have been published are described. (If there are others out there, I'd like to know about them for my next book!). The earliest comfort experiment was done by Hogan-Miller, Rustad, Sendelbach, and Goldenberg (1995), followed by two experiments that I conducted and published. Lastly, I will describe a fascinating study that a doctoral student/midwife is doing to assess the existence of comfort in labor and delivery. I will also demonstrate how to start literally with line 4 in Figure 5.2, reprinted below for this chapter as Figure 7.1. Line 4 is the mid-range theory level and includes the three types of health seeking behaviors (HSBs) identified by Schlotfeldt (1975). Through substruction, variables in line 4 are specified for your patients and/or your research setting. After starting with line 4, every comfort study can and should have unique versions of lines 5 and 6, as depicted in this chapter.

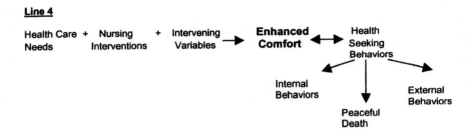

Line 4

FIGURE 7.1   Mid-Range Theory of Comfort.

CONCEPTUAL AND OPERATIONAL DEFINITIONS OF COMFORT

As stated at the end of chapter 6, exploring the defining attributes of patient comfort enabled us to become clear on the boundaries of its technical definition. From this precise definition, embodied in the taxonomic structure (TS), we generated conceptual and operational definitions of comfort. *Conceptual definitions* are statements about the meanings of words in plain language. The technical definition of comfort (see below) is, at the same time, a conceptual definition because comfort is defined in plain words, but in a more complicated and precise way than a layperson would do. For example, in the breast cancer study where I was addressing Total Comfort, my conceptual (technical) definition of comfort was: a desired outcome achieved when needs for Relief, Ease, and Transcendence are met within physical, social, psychospiritual, and environmental contexts (Kolcaba & Fox, 1999).

Operational definitions are ways in which the researcher decides to measure the concept, usually in the form of questionnaires, interviews, or scales. Most studies have more than one operational definition for each concept of interest, which enhances construct validity. My breast cancer study utilized the RTCQ and four VASs to measure comfort. These instruments comprised the operational definitions for comfort in the breast cancer study.

The important thing to remember here is that both types of definitions (conceptual and operational) are essential for testing theoretical relationships between concepts. Of course, all concepts pertaining to the research problem that you want to measure must have conceptual and operational definitions. Your theoretical framework will help you achieve congruence between the two types of definitions. If you want to design a comfort study using the theoretical framework that I find useful, remember that line 4 is the abstract, theoretical level and it depicts the Mid-Range Theory of Comfort. Line 5, which I will construct for each of the studies described below, is a more concrete level naming the variables of interest for each specific research setting. Each variable in line 5 should have its own conceptual definition accompanying the diagram. Line 6 shows how the variables are going to be measured in your study. It is the most concrete level in your diagram. Each variable in line 6 should have its own operational definition, or name of an instrument, accompanying the diagram. In any given comfort study, parts or all of the Mid-Range Theory can be tested.

Thus, in each of my descriptions of the experiments below, I will add specific diagrams that show how lines 5 and 6 guided that study. This is done to demonstrate that, by adhering rigorously to your own diagram (theoretical framework), you will be more likely to design an efficient, thoughtful study, that doesn't waste the time and energy of your research participants, and that produces significant results. My hope is that, if you are armed with knowledge about the intuitive nature of comfort studies and their probability for success, *you* will bring to fruition a new generation of comfort studies.

FOUR QUANTITATIVE STUDIES

1. Hogan-Miller et al. (1995)—Effects of Three Methods of Femoral Site Mobilization on Bleeding and Comfort After Coronary Angiogram

This study has the distinction of being the first comfort study using the TS of comfort, and the one that I believe helped spur editors to publish the TS article (Kolcaba, 1991). As I mentioned in chapter 3, Elaine Hogan-Miller was an experienced clinical researcher who spoke to me about her then-current research after I presented the TS at a regional research conference. Hogan-Miller was working with post-angiogram patients who were immobilized for 6 hours after their procedure in order to prevent femoral site bleeding. While they were not in pain, the required immobilization caused these patients to be decidedly uncomfortable. Their muscles were stiff, the environment was nerve-wracking, they were anxious about the results of their angiogram, they were hungry and thirsty, they needed to void, they were restless, etc. These were the types of discomforts that I was talking about in my presentation, which were very different from pain. Moreover, one discomfort enhanced other discomforts, so this was a holistically uncomfortable, but not painful, experience for patients.

Hogan-Miller was aware of three types of immobilization methods that were being used in practice: the use of sandbags, sheet restraints, and verbal instructions. She wanted to test which method was best in terms of patient comfort and hemostasis. She was also aware of other patient factors that could affect the outcomes, such as body mass, gender, age, weight, extent of coronary artery disease, length of procedure, and type and amount of anticoagulants and pain medication. Her dilemma was how to consider these factors in her research design and what to use to measure comfort in a population where pain was not the issue.

After our discussion, I drew a diagram similar to that depicted in Figure 7.2 to help organize my thinking as her "comfort consultant." Hogan-Miller and I discussed limiting the comfort instrument to physical and psychological comfort, to reduce patient burden. (This issue of length I usually leave up to the clinician when I am not familiar with the patient population.) Hogan-Miller and I wrote 38 items that covered physical and psychological comfort in the ease and relief senses. A pilot study of this instrument with 30 angiogram patients resulted in a coefficient alpha of .73, which is in the moderate range for a new instrument. Under pressure from her fellow nurses, who thought an instrument with 38 items was too long, the instrument was reduced further to 19 physical items. It is important to note here, however, that her coefficient alpha using the shorter instrument, was about the same in the study with 188 angiogram patients as it was in the pilot (.74 at Time 1 and .67 at Time 2 in the full study). Therefore, from my perspective, Hogan-Miller lost a great deal of information about psychological comfort and its effect on physical comfort and achieved little gain by shortening the instrument.

Hogan-Miller limited her definition of comfort to physical comfort because that was what she decided to measure. She defined physical comfort as pertaining to bodily sensations where human needs for Ease, Relief, and Transcendence are met (Hogan-Miller et al., 1995). She used a 19-item Bedrest Comfort Questionnaire to measure physical

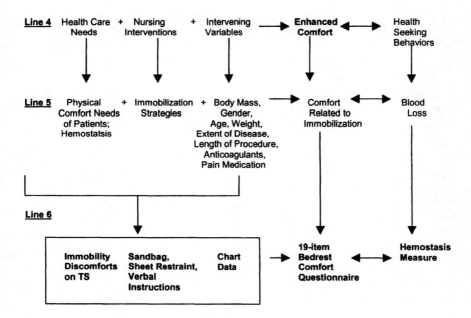

FIGURE 7.2 Theoretical framework for coronary angiography study.
Note: Boldface indicates operational variables measured in this study (Hogan-Miller et al., 1995).

comfort. In this study, her conceptual and operational definitions matched her research problem.

Hemostasis was measured by an instrument created for this study. It was a rating by nurses from 1 (signifying no bleeding or hematoma) to 5 (signifying bleeding significant enough to require surgical intervention). This instrument had an inter-rater reliability of 100% agreement between two data collectors in a pilot test with five patients.

Effectiveness of each immobilization method was measured through random assignment of patients to one of the three methods immediately after the angiogram and subsequent mandatory application of manual pressure. All of the intervening variables were assessed when looking at differences between groups at Time 1, a step that is important to do prior to analyzing the data. No significant differences were identified for any of the intervening variables listed in Figure 7.2, and Hogan-Miller concluded that her groups were similar at baseline. Also, we were mindful that the study period would be limited to the 6 hours in which patients were immobilized. Thus, two data collection points were used for measurements of comfort and hemostasis from all participants in the three groups, at 2–3 hours and 5–6 hours post-angiogram.

The findings of this research were that the verbal instruction group bled the most and because of the high number of bleeding incidences, this group was not included in the analysis of comfort among the groups. The analysis of variance on group differences in comfort between the restraint and sandbag groups revealed a significance level of $p = .0689$. This almost approached the selected alpha of .05, the traditional Cronbach's alpha used as a cutoff to decide whether there are statistically significant differences between groups.

Post-angiographic bleeding was conceptualized as a health seeking behavior (HSB) by me, because it fits Schlotfeldt's definition of an internal HSB (1975). By putting it in the theoretical framework as a subsequent outcome to comfort, I hypothesized that patients who are most comfortable will have the least amount of postoperative bleeding. This may sound like a stretch, but think about factors associated with acute discomfort, such as squirming, hypertension, muscular tension, and anxiety that could promote bleeding. Elaine did not report which of the three groups was most comfortable, but if she had, the above hypothesis could be tested.

2. Kolcaba & Fox (1999)—The Effects of Guided Imagery on Comfort of Women with Early Stage Breast Cancer Undergoing Radiation Therapy

In chapters 1 and 2, I wrote about the human side of my comfort quest, with my goal being to complete and successfully defend my dissertation. As you might recall, my dissertation study was an experiment that was designed to show how nurses could enhance patients' comfort over time, given an effective and repetitive intervention. In this chapter, I will describe the study more objectively and succinctly, so that all the information is in one place and uncluttered by personal elements.

The research problem that I identified for my dissertation was how to enhance comfort in women who were recently diagnosed with early-stage breast cancer (usually a devastating event) and who had chosen breast conserving therapy to treat their cancer. Breast conserving therapy consisted of local excision of the tumor, followed by radiation therapy (RT) for a usual 6-week course of therapy with a booster dose of radiation afterward. Because only 5% of breast cancers occur in males, this study was limited to women.

The study follows the theoretical framework depicted in Figure 7.3. Comfort needs of this population were many and were described in popular magazine articles, descriptive nursing journal articles, books by cancer survivors, newspaper series, etc. From these sources, comfort needs were identified and organized on a TS. Because the needs were conceptualized holistically, an intervention was designed that could address these needs in a systematic and holistic way.

Guided imagery (GI) was the intervention that I chose, because it could be scripted to address the identified needs and it could be deliv-

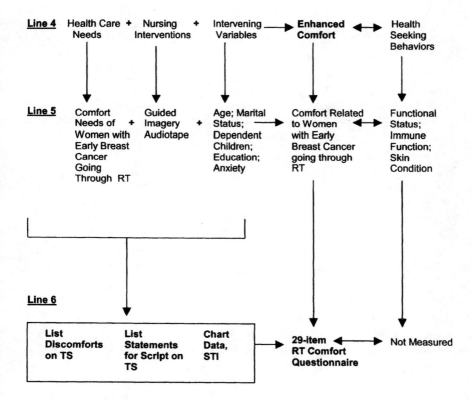

FIGURE 7.3 Theoretical framework for breast cancer/radiation therapy (RT) study.

Note: Boldface indicates operational variables measured in this study (Kolcaba & Fox, 1999).

ered on an audiotape every day at the women's convenience. The intervention began prior to RT. Daily repetition of the intervention was important in order to be able to demonstrate a trend for increased comfort over time compared to a control group.

I wrote the main part of the script for the GI intervention, and I targeted the comfort needs of my population as organized on the TS. In the script, RT was reframed as a "friend" whose healing rays were important for the women's health. Each sentence spoke to one or several comfort needs. For example, the statement, "The large machinery is helpful to you as you work to return to good health," addressed psychospiritual and environmental comfort, whereas the statement, "The table is a reassuring presence, providing strong support for your body, holding you firmly as you receive the healing rays," addressed social, environmental, and psychospiritual comfort (Kolcaba & Fox, 1999). A professional GI practitioner, who had recorded and marketed several of her own GI tapes, was hired to record the tape. She chose soothing background music and scripted the induction and waking up phases of the GI. (An extensive literature review about GI was also presented in my dissertation about the principles behind composing and recording a meaningful audiotape [Kolcaba, 1998].) Since I did most of the data collection, I did not record the tape; the voice of someone they knew might have influenced the women's responses to the tape.

There were several possible intervening variables, such as age, marital status, number of dependent children, education, and anxiety. If the groups were different on any of these variables at baseline, those variables would be used as covariates. The State Anxiety Inventory (Spielberger, 1983) was used to measure anxiety prior to beginning RT. Data about the other variables were obtained from the demographic sheet.

To measure comfort, I adapted the General Comfort Questionnaire (GCQ) for my population of women with early-stage breast cancer. After deleting items from the GCQ that were not relevant, I placed the remaining questions on the TS and filled in the holes with new questions specific to my breast cancer study. New questions were derived from the popular and scientific literature and from interviews with breast cancer survivors and RT personnel, including nurses, technicians, and physicians. There were an even number of positive and negative questions. As a result of this process, the Radiation Therapy Comfort Questionnaire (RTCQ) had 26 questions with a six-response Likert-type format, ranging from "strongly disagree" to "strongly agree." Higher scores indicated higher comfort in a range of 26 to 156. For this population, Cronbach's alpha was .76, indicating moderate reliability for a new instrument. The RTCQ is reprinted in Appendix B, and is available in Cumulative Index of Nursing and Allied Health Literature (CINAHL) and through my web pages (Kolcaba, online).

Visual analog scales also were constructed to measure Total Comfort, Relief, Ease, and Transcendence, but I did not report the results in my first dissertation article, because much secondary analysis of the data had to be conducted and interpreted. (A full discussion and analysis of the data that the VAS produced takes place in chapter 4.)

Three measurement points were chosen that I hoped would demonstrate differences in comfort over time. To obtain the baseline measurement that is essential in experiments, the comfort questionnaires were completed before the RT and the intervention started (Time 1). The second measurement took place in the middle of therapy (Time 2), and the third measurement occurred 3 weeks after RT was completed (Time 3). Decisions about when to measure comfort were based on the literature and on consultations with nurses at the RT departments. The 3-week interval between times 1 and 2 was chosen because this would allow time for GI to make a difference. My third time point, 3 weeks after RT was completed, was selected because the literature review revealed that this was often a time of high anxiety for this population (Kolcaba & Fox, 1999).

I provided the women in both groups with small tape players that they could clip to their clothing, a suggestion from the RT technicians who thought some women might listen to the tape during RT. Women in the control group received a different audiotape at the end of the study that emphasized health and had been previously recorded by my GI consultant. At the end of the study, women could keep the tape and tape player, or they could choose a cash incentive of $20.00. Most women chose to keep their tape and tape player. Funding for the study was requested and received from my Alumni Association at CWRU, from two chapters of Sigma Theta Tau with which I was affiliated, and from the American Nurses Foundation.

The convenience sample consisted of 53 women from two RT departments in the Midwest. Eligibility criteria were that women were (a) 17 years of age or older, (b) fluent in English, (c) had adequate hearing for listening to the audiotape, (d) diagnosed with Stage I or II breast cancer, and (e) about to begin RT. Those with previous malignancies, prior experience with GI, or psychological disorders (as determined by chart review or interview) were excluded. Random assignment resulted in 26 women in the treatment group and 27 women in the comparison group. Nurses from the RT departments introduced the study to eligible candidates during their pre-simulation appointment. Names and phone numbers of women who were interested in the study were forwarded to me or my second data collector, and we contacted the women immediately. The design of the study required baseline data to be gathered prior to the beginning of RT and the intervention.

Alpha was set at .10 because the intervention had no risks and the higher alpha reduced Type II error (Lipsey, 1990). Analysis of group differences in demographic data and anxiety revealed that the groups were similar for all of these variables. This analysis was one of the assumptions we tested before proceeding with Repeated Measures Multivariate Analysis of Variance (RM MANOVA). This test statistic was conducted on group data at three time points to capture interaction effects between the groups and time. The F value was .07, which meant that there were significant differences between the groups on comfort when looking at all the data. Then my statistician and I did two posttests. The first was to determine which group had higher comfort (the treatment group did at the second and third time points) and the second was to perform a trend analysis, looking at the slopes of the comfort data for both groups when plotted on a line by the computer. This analysis revealed a linear slope over time, meaning that the differences between groups increased steadily when considering the interaction effects. A simplified picture of the trend analysis for this study is presented in Figure 7.4.

This was the best outcome I could have hoped for, because it supported the original theory from Murray (chapter 5), captured in his concept of unitary trend. Murray (1938) stated that given a successful intervention over time, a trend for a positive perception of the experience could be achieved. (If experiences were negative, a negative trend could be another result.) The linear trend demonstrated in Figure 7.4 gave empirical support to Murray's notion that efforts to intervene in a stressful stimulus situation can be successful. Note the importance of linking your study to an existing theoretical perspective—it gives you direction and insight!

My dissertation study was limited to testing the first part of Comfort Theory in Figure 7.3, the bolded variables. That is, nurses and/or members of the health care team address known comfort needs by designing interventions that target those needs. If repeated often enough and if pleasing, a trend for increased comfort can be demon-

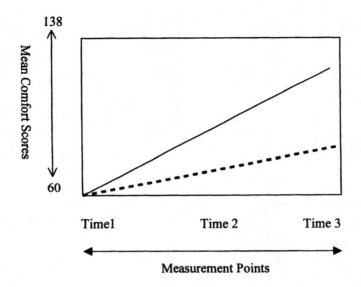

FIGURE 7.4 Trend analysis for breast cancer study.
Treatment group = solid line; Comparison group = dotted line.
Source: Kolcaba & Fox, 1999.

strated, even though comfort is state-specific. As suggested in Figure 7.3, this study could have gone further by testing the relationships between the immediate outcome of enhanced comfort and subsequent health seeking behaviors such as functional status, immune function, and/or stress. Thus, all or parts of the Theory of Comfort can be tested at one time, or in an extended program of research.

3. Dowd, Kolcaba, & Steiner (2000)—Using Cognitive Strategies to Enhance Bladder Control and Comfort

The purpose of this study was to test the effectiveness of audiotaped cognitive strategies for improving bladder function and comfort related to bladder function. Urinary incontinence (UI) was the research program of the first author, Dr. Therese Dowd. She approached me with the suggestion that we blend our programs of research because her qualitative research had revealed many holistic comfort needs associated with UI. Dowd also had an interest in cognitive strategies (CS) because her psychologist-husband had developed many of the techniques associated with this psychotherapeutic technique (Dowd & Dowd, 1995).

Following our theoretical framework (depicted in Figure 7.5), we organized the known comfort needs of this population and designed statements for our audiotaped CS using the TS as a guide. We looked at age, gender, and particulars of bladder health history for our possible covariates (intervening variables). To measure comfort in this population, we used the TS to develop the Urinary Incontinence and Frequency Comfort Questionnaire (UIFCQ) and we pilot tested it prior to using it in this study. Our health seeking behavior was improved bladder

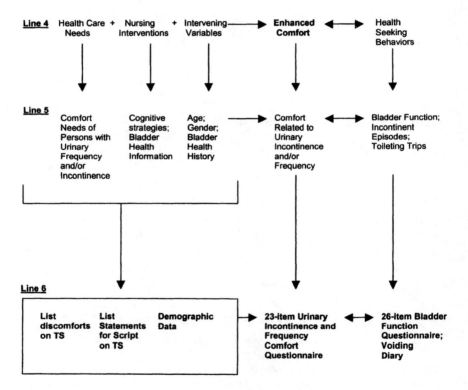

FIGURE 7.5 Theoretical framework for study of cognitive strategies to enhance bladder control and comfort.

Note: Boldface indicates operational variables measured in this study (Dowd, Kolcaba, & Steiner, 2000).

function as measured by the Bladder Function Questionnaire, a second instrument that we developed and pilot tested prior to this study. Bladder function was also conceptualized by number of incontinent episodes and number of toileting trips.

We borrowed most of the methods that I developed in my breast cancer study (described previously), including having persons in the treatment group listen to an audiotape daily, having three data collection points, and using the same method of data analysis.

Results indicated that the treatment group had more comfort and improved bladder function compared with the comparison group (Dowd, Kolcaba, & Steiner, 2000). (The UIFCQ is reprinted in this article; we were denied permission to reprint it elsewhere.) In addition, we added a crossover component and asked those in the original comparison group to listen to the audiotape for 3 weeks, after which we collected data at time 4 for both groups. We found a significant improvement of bladder function in the crossover group and their comfort had increased to the level of the treatment group after 3 weeks of the intervention.

Another interesting finding was that the UIFCQ predicted the participants (n = 17, or 90% of the treatment group) who demonstrated improvement in incontinence. Thus, comfort was a strong predictor of who benefits from treatment for incontinence and frequency, supporting the Mid-Range Theory of Comfort (Dowd, Kolcaba, & Steiner, 2000). This study was funded by the Ohio Kidney Foundation.

In a subsequent study (Dowd, Kolcaba, & Steiner, 2002), we wanted to determine the predictive properties for comfort, the immediate outcome, on our subsequent outcomes (HSBs) which were perception of health, bladder function, and episodes of urinary frequency and incontinence. We found that comfort was moderately related in the expected directions to bladder function (R = .52), to perception of health (R = .40), to urinary frequency (R = −.40), and to incontinent episodes (R = −.21). The latter two correlations are interpreted that as comfort increases, urinary frequency and incontinence decrease. These findings supported our earlier findings that comfort is a predictor of HSBs and that a recursive relationship between comfort and HSBs exists. Path analysis would provide us with more information about which variable (comfort or a specific HSB) comes first. There was no path analysis done in this study, however, because there were not enough subjects.

4. Schuiling (dissertation, in press)—Identifying the Physiologic Path of Comforting Interventions: Focus on Childbirth

This is a fascinating study begun by a nurse-midwife who published an earlier article about the "radical" idea of comfort in labor and delivery (Schuiling & Sampselle, 1999). After the publication of her article, I congratulated Schuiling on her ideas about comfort being a transcendent and strengthening force for the rigors of maternal labor. She told me she was pursuing her PhD at the University of Michigan, and asked me to be the outside member on her dissertation committee, to which I readily agreed. So began a long and fruitful relationship for both of us.

In her dissertation study, Schuiling wants to quantify the existence of comfort during labor and delivery (L&D), thus providing empirical evidence for her previously published theoretical ideas. The theoretical framework in Figure 7.6 is mine and I have used it to help Schuiling design her instrument and her methods (Schuiling has designed her own conceptual framework with comfort in it). Following the figure, the comfort needs of women in L&D will be identified. Comfort in women delivering their babies will be assessed and, as a result of their responses on the comfort questionnaire, will be divided into two groups. One group will be those who score above the mean and the other group will be those who score below the mean. On comfort interventions, social support, and amount and type of pain medication will be important intervening variables.

Schuiling designed a 14-item comfort questionnaire following the TS and she will administer it at baseline, before L&D commences, during the intermediate stages of L&D, and at transition. She will analyze her data with RM MANCOVA if there are covariates and RM MANOVA if there are no covariates. For her dissertation, Schuiling hopes that the psychometric properties of her questionnaire are strong, the women in active labor are able to answer the questionnaire, and the questionnaire is sensitive to differences between the groups. These outcomes will form the base for her program of research. Later, she hopes to test a theoretical link between enhanced comfort and decreased perineal damage.

WHAT WE LEARNED FROM THE ABOVE STUDIES

Congruence

Theoretical frameworks are invaluable for designing studies that are congruent from top to bottom. If you are interested in designing a

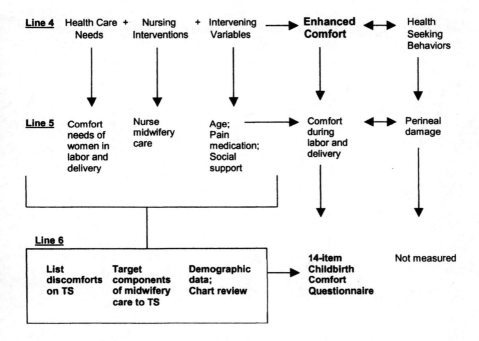

FIGURE 7.6 Theoretical framework for study of comfort during labor and delivery.

Note: Boldface indicates operational variables measured in this study (Schuiling, in press).

comfort study, please keep in mind that this framework works best for whole-person needs and interventions. This is common thread throughout the studies discussed in this chapter. Interestingly, the contacts I have received about other comfort studies contain this thread as well. For example, one graduate student was most earnest about designing a music therapy tape for burn unit patients undergoing dressing changes. Another nurse researcher was doing life-flight nursing, and was concerned about the holistic comfort of patients during emergency transport. Yet another nurse wanted to enhance the comfort of women going through gynecological examinations. These, and the studies in this chapter, are examples of whole-person patient stress in health care situations and they all seem to speak to the mediation of diverse, but interrelated, uncomfortable experiences that do not necessarily involve a lot of physical pain.

Significant results are most likely when your intervention is targeted specifically to your patients' needs, and where the items on your holistic comfort questionnaire are congruent with the comfort needs of your patients and your intervention. Intervening variables must be explicated for consideration in your methods section: Will you deal with them by design or analysis? Subsequent outcomes and relevant health seeking behaviors, and/or institutional outcomes (see chapter 9) also must be congruent with the population, research problems, interventions, group differences, and research questions. Constructing your own theoretical framework guides you in making these crucial decisions, in writing about those decisions for funding or publication, and for talking through the study with auxiliary personnel and/or faculty.

Alpha

As discussed earlier, when selecting your cutoff level for determining whether your findings are significant, please consider the advice of Lipsey (1990) who has some insights for researchers in the social sciences. He believes that in much of the human science research, interventions or natural groups carry very little risk. My guided imagery intervention is an example of a treatment that, even if it doesn't have the desired effect on patient comfort isn't going to hurt anyone. Therefore, why not relax the alpha a bit from the stringent .05 level that is geared toward preventing a Type I error? A Type I error is committed when we think that an intervention achieved significance, but it actually did not. You do *not* want to commit Type I error when doing drug trials, for example, because this error would cause potentially harmful medications to be given in the future, thinking that they "worked" for facilitating a specified health outcome. Therefore, for interventions that have risk, it is good to prevent Type I error.

If we relax alpha to .10, however, we are showing that we are also concerned about committing a Type II error, which happens when we think our findings are not significant when they actually are. I would have committed a Type II error if the alpha for my guided imagery intervention was set at the traditional .05 level. An F value of .07, which was obtained in that study, would not have achieved significance and the intervention might have been dropped from the repertoire of successful, easy-to-administer interventions.

Lipsey believes that one reason many of the early human science experimental studies were reported as having nonsignificant findings, is that their alphas were too stringent for the degree of risk entailed in the intervention. He suggests that we attempt to achieve a balance between Type I and Type II error, based on the degree of risk that the intervention entails. For most holistic interventions, such as art, music therapy, or bubble-blowing as a pediatric distraction, we should make the adjustment toward preventing Type II error with a less stringent alpha of .10. For interventions with potential risks, such as medications, the traditional alpha of .05 is more appropriate. Remember, an alpha of .10 is still respectful of Type I error, just not overly so.

Test Statistic

Another thing that we learned from the studies above is that statistics can be a holistic art. We really like RM MANCOVA or RM MANOVA (depending on whether or not covariates are present) because they capture interaction effects between time and interventions, and this is congruent with our holistic paradigm. When I was making these decisions about my dissertation studies, most MANOVAS were run with more than two groups. That's what made them "multivariate." My creative statisticians, however, following Stevens's text (1992) which I had been using, also used MANOVAS to measure differences between two groups over time—that is, using more than two measurement points. Hence, all of my studies have at least three measurement points. This methodological solution was especially congruent with Comfort Theory, which looked at whole-person responses over time. By looking at all the data at once, from two or more groups, the test statistic RM MANCOVA captures interaction effects between interventions and time, which is what holism is all about.

Bias

The above studies, and any experimental study done in the human sciences, are biased by the self-selection of the research participants. We know in our breast cancer study that about half of the women who were informed about their eligibility to participate in the study, actually chose to do so. The rest were either too terrified about their diagnosis to add another activity to their plate, or they did not believe that GI would help them, or they had no energy to be proactive in enhancing their own comfort. So the women who participated in our study consciously *chose* to try to enhance their comfort.

Likewise, in the urinary incontinence study, persons from the community who self-selected to be in the study *chose* to try the intervention in order to enhance their comfort but also to try to improve their bladder function. They chose to go beyond their comfort zone, in which they wore incontinence pads and accepted their incontinence as a "normal" sequelae of aging or childbirth.

Thus, the choices that our research participants make bias our studies. We are tapping into people who are oriented to finding better ways to live, who are open-minded, who seek to manage their stress constructively. An important question remaining is this: How do we comfort those who do not make their needs known or who do not believe long-term health interventions fit their lives? Are their comfort zones (baseline) different from those who seek comfort more overtly?

MUSINGS ON COMFORT QUOTE (CHAPTER 7)

> They knew luxury, they knew beggary, but they never knew *comfort*.
> —Samuel Johnson, 1750
> (letter about making a living through writing)

Here, we see that people in very different situations can share some types of discomfort. Some writers live in luxury, where all of their physical needs are met. Others live in poverty and have unmet needs for safety, food, and shelter. What they have in common, though, is their longing to write something meaningful and enduring. This longing can be a major discomfort that can't be alleviated, even when in the process of actively writing, and this discomfort is more important than their situational circumstances.

Needing to fulfill one's goals (dare we say destiny) is a gnawing and constant urge that prevents complete ease and can rarely be relieved, except by transcending the barriers and working toward one's goals. If we choose to listen to this motivating force, we will move outside of our comfort zones whether the goal is rehabilitation, remission, or some other personal achievement. Not everyone chooses to do this or has the resources to do this. But being in our comfort zones provides respite and *strengthens* us for the fight.

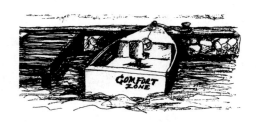

CHAPTER 8

The Ethics of Comfort Care*

> I made a finer end, and he went away as if he had been any Christian child. He parted just between twelve and one, for after I saw him fumble with the sheets, and play with flowers, and smile upon his fingers' end, I knew there was but one way. . . . "How now, Sir John! What, man, be of good cheer." So he cried out, "God, God, God!" three or four times. Now I, to comfort him, bid him he should not think of God; I hoped there was no need to trouble himself with any such thought yet. So he bade me lay more clothes on his feet; I put my hand into the bed and felt them, and they were as cold as any stone.
> —William Shakespeare (~1598), *King Henry the Fifth*, Act 2, Scene 3 (Death scene of Falstaff as told by Hostess Quigley)

Recently, my husband and I received an invitation to present The Ethics of Comfort Care at the Midwest Meeting of The American Philosophical Association. We had not developed this topic before, although it certainly fits well with our interests in decision making and end-of-life issues. Before accepting, though, we reviewed how the study of ethics is organized. This chapter utilizes that organizational scheme to frame the discussion about Comfort Care and to merge it

---

*This chapter written in collaboration with Dr. Raymond Kolcaba.

with three aspects of ethics that deal with making choices. Case studies and the comfort quote above augment the discussions.

THE STUDY OF ETHICS

Ethics is the study of conduct, and conduct is chosen behavior. In the standard case, choice stems from a special kind of thinking called deliberation. We deliberate about alternatives open to us by weighing them. We then determine the best alternative and choose it. The study of ethics can be divided into three aspects of the deliberative process. We can employ principles of conduct in our deliberations. This has sometimes been called the ethics of obligation. We can utilize estimates of the consequences of proposed actions to weigh alternatives. The action that promises the best consequences (outcomes) is judged to be right. This has been termed consequentialist ethics. The character traits of the person deliberating assist in reasoning and motivating action. This has been called the ethics of virtue.

Ethics of Obligation

The basis of the ethics of obligation is common morality. This is what parents teach children as the difference between right and wrong. The aim of such teaching is for children to develop a moral sense or conscience. The intellectual side of moral sense is expressed as a group of rules or principles. Examples from common morality include that one ought not lie, one ought not cheat, and one ought to keep one's promises. The emotional side of moral sense is moral psychology. It involves feelings like responsibility, guilt, shame, and duty. Moral psychology guides our use of moral principles.

Beyond common morality we find other rules such as laws and codes of professional conduct. Within nursing, we have a code of ethics for all nurses (Appendix G), principles embodied in theories of practice, and standards of care relative to specialties such as gerontology or hospice. Legal obligations and professional obligations are created through the application of these rules to practical situations. Other disciplines associated with health care have their codes of ethics as well.

Consequentialist Ethics

Choice and action are productive. They bring about change. Change can be to ourselves, others, or the world around us. When we ask what choice to make, we are asking what changes are desirable. The simple answer is, "Those that are good." The philosopher then asks, "What is good?" We raise the question of value. A consequentialist ethic develops a view of what is good. Actions are right or morally preferred if they bring about the best consequences. In other words, actions are right or wrong based on results of those actions.

A significant portion of nursing thought is directed toward desirable patient outcomes. Therapeutic decisions are based on promised results. The treatment that brings about the best results is taken to be ethically the best choice. For example, if we want to justify giving a patient morphine, we may do so by claiming that it has the desirable consequence of relieving pain and has few side effects.

Virtue Ethics

A virtue is a positive character state. Wisdom, courage, and honesty are common virtues. A character state consists of a disposition. The wise person is disposed to act wisely, the courageous person to act courageously, and the honest person to act honestly. The disposition is to having a feeling. The honest person feels honest. The feeling serves as a motivator for honest action. When we judge that a person is honest in character, we know that it is predictive—we expect that the person will act honestly.

The prototype nurse possesses a certain kind of character. We may pick out certain virtues as typifying nurses, such as caring, compassionate, sympathetic, optimistic, and so on. Such a person is disposed to feel "like a nurse"; the person possesses the right character states or virtues to be a nurse.

Comfort Care and Supererogation

When discussing the ethics of Comfort Care, we notice how ethics of obligation, consequence, and virtue are brought together. The ethics of nursing is usually approached through an ethics of obligation: common morality joined to other legal and professional codes. In practice, obligations specify duties. Duties indicate what nurses owe their patients. Patients have rights to certain care based on those duties. Nurses are doing their job well if those rights are fulfilled. Exactly what nurses are *obligated* to do is spelled out in job descriptions and codes of ethics prepared by professional organizations such as the American Nurses Association and the International Council of Nurses (Appendixes G and H). You will note that neither set of codes make mention of virtues such as compassion or beneficence. Goodness of character is not addressed.

Comfort Care, however, goes beyond duty. It is supererogatory. This does not mean that nurses must make self-sacrifices. It means that Comfort Care supplements what is required by duty. Supererogatory acts can involve extreme sacrifice but they don't have to; they can involve simply saying a few kind words to a victim who was hit by a car. The boundary of supererogation is not the extremity of the act but where duty leaves off. Duty can require danger and risk of harm; the duties of firefighters are such. The dispatcher who gives a child money for ice cream also acts beyond the call of duty. The extent of supererogation possible, then, depends upon the limits of obligation. Comprehensive obligations leave little room for supererogation while few obligations leave much room for it.

The exercise of supererogatory virtues is often described as "above and beyond the call of duty." The call of duty implies that one is performing the obligations of their profession within its principles, rules, standards, and codes. The phrase "beyond the call of duty" brings to mind virtue traits such as extreme bravery, great dedication, extraordinary compassion, heroic leadership, and high regard for others. When nurses rush to hurricane sites to help in shelters and render first aid and comfort, they leave their own families and homes sometimes for weeks. Clearly, such nurses demonstrate action beyond what is expected and beyond what most of us feel we can do.

COMFORT CARE ACROSS HEALTH DISCIPLINES

In 1995, I defined Comfort Care as "a nursing art that entails the process of comforting actions performed by a nurse for a patient and the outcome of enhanced comfort that is brought into being" (Kolcaba, 1995b, p. 288). Enhanced comfort is desirable because, by further definition, it strengthens patients to engage in health seeking behaviors, such as going through rehabilitation, chemotherapy, or medical problems. It can also strengthen patients (and families) to make decisions that will facilitate a peaceful death (Kolcaba & Fisher, 1996).

Although the idea of Comfort Care began in nursing, it is a theoretical perspective that can be adopted and applied in many disciplines that interface in health care, such as theology, social work, medicine, and psychology. The term Comfort Care is a dynamic combination of two terms, comfort and care. The terms work together to provide an image of health-related support where comfort is the goal (noun) *and* the type of health care delivered (adjective). The term care is expressed as close attention to patients (noun) *and* as an action word (verb). Thus, providers using this framework perform actions that express caring for each patient for the specific immediate goal of enhancing their comfort.

Comfort Care entails keen attention to physical comfort needs, expressed or unexpressed. Some unmet physical needs may be related to medical problems such as needs for adequate or normalized oxygenation, fluid balance, immune response, nutrition, ventilation, mobility, blood chemistries, elimination, et cetera. Sometimes these acute physical needs take priority over other comfort needs (psychospiritual, sociocultural, and environmental). However, all needs should be addressed, often bringing about a healthier, holistic response in the physical realm. In this broad and proactive context, Comfort Care is appropriate for most health care settings, providers, and populations of patients, including families and groups.

Advantages of Comfort Care include its being humanistic, empowering, individualistic, goal directed, and beneficial to institutions that promote it. It can be an interdisciplinary framework because it fits within the ethical structure of health care principles and common morality across disciplines. Comfort Care directs all health-related disciplines to focus on decisions for each patient that will enhance his or her comfort; thus it is a unifying model. Ideally, Comfort Care is intentional and disciplines must value patient comfort in order to make decisions to promote comfort. Comfort Care also provides us with a framework for going "beyond the call of duty."

Comfort Care is simple and intuitive to learn and practice because, regardless of background, we are familiar with our own comfort needs, how they interact with each other, how they can be assuaged, and the benefits of "feeling comfortable." Comfort Care melds nicely with other ethical values in health care, thereby fitting into a wider patient care ethic. The ethical categories of obligations, consequences, and virtues serve to organize the remainder of the chapter.

ETHICAL OBLIGATIONS

Beneficence

Throughout this book, I have stated strongly that Comfort Care is of value to patients—it is what they want and hope for from their nurses and other team members. Therefore, Comfort Care has altruistic properties—it is pleasant for patients and they feel better when they receive it. Providers who practice Comfort Care are demonstrating an ethic of beneficence, or an ethic of "doing nice things" because they ought to be done. Following this ethic, comfort is a worthy end or goal unto itself.

Beneficence is part of the common morality of the health care profession. We are directed first to do no harm, and second to do good. A shortcoming of this ethic, however, is its generality. We ask the question, "What beneficent acts count as being professional obligations and what count as going beyond the call of duty?" Because the boundaries of professional obligations have not been made explicit, staff and managerial cuts have narrowed the possibilities for nurses and team members to practice routinely at the high end of beneficence. Most nurses want to practice at their best, and being unable to do so has frustrated nurses and diminished patient satisfaction with care.

Therefore, a related shortcoming of the ethic of beneficence is that it is resource related. That is, when health care providers do not have time, administrative encouragement, or reimbursement for doing "nice things," these actions are sacrificed for more obvious and immediate professional obligations. Sadly, comfort as a sufficient and desirable consequence for patients is a low priority for many institutional administrators. By demonstrating that comfort has a strong relationship with health or other outcomes of interest, however, nurses may be able to convince administrators to give Comfort Care a higher priority.

As discussed in chapter 9, most administrators want to know whether patient comfort (and the augmented staff that increased patient comfort might require) has concrete payoffs, beyond conforming to an ethic of beneficence. For example, they might want to see an increase in patient satisfaction (compared to an institution that did not have an augmented staff), or an improvement in the bottom line (resulting from decreased length of stay or readmission). In short, an ethic of beneficence for its own sake is not currently a high priority in our capitalistic society and health care system—but we can change that, with our vision of creating a health care system that values patient comfort!

Autonomy

Comfort Care adds another ethical dimension to patient care, beyond beneficence. Comfort Care is based on patients' needs and patients' input about their needs. When their needs are addressed, patients are strengthened. So, Comfort Care is an empowering and motivating force for patients when they need and want to make decisions or act in their own interests. It helps patients "get through" crises, hardships, and unwanted but necessary treatments and/or rehabilitation. It helps patients die peacefully, when that is the most realistic goal. Thus, in alert and legally competent patients, Comfort Care encourages patients' autonomy (self-determination).

However, there are inherent burdens with autonomy in the health care arena. Those burdens include the need for complete information from several sources. The gathering of information central to the decision(s) at hand takes time, energy, education, money, connections, computer and library skills, and perseverance. Second opinions require permission from insurance companies. These burdens are exacerbated by the stressors of unexpected pathology or illness, when patients or their family members are under extreme duress and pressure to make decisions quickly. Thus, in health care, patient autonomy (like free enterprise) is often unrealistic.

There are other deterrents to autonomy in health care. These include (a) patients' adherence to cultural practices that emphasize group norms over self-determination; (b) patients' or family members' socialization into subservient or passive roles; (c) lack of background or will to put pieces of information together in meaningful ways; and (d) an attitude of trust or loyalty for specific health care providers. For example, my mother doesn't want to hurt the feelings of her health providers by going elsewhere, even when it is clear that her care is substandard. Moreover, patient autonomy is not appropriate for infants and small children, comatose patients, or patients with cognitive impairment due to trauma or disease.

Because of these factors and a general orientation to vitality, invulnerability, and denial of death, only 10%–20% of adults in this country have signed advance directives. This may be surprising in view of the passage of the Patient Self-Determination Act in 1990 (Robinson, 2001). Should the 80% plus adults without advance directives be suddenly unable to make decisions about their health care, someone else would have to make choices for them. That someone else might be a loved one, acting on what they think the patient would want, or in some cases, a physician who doesn't know the patient. The framework of Comfort Care offers guidelines for these scenarios as well, which philosophers call situations of *entrusted care*.

ETHICAL CONSEQUENCES OF ENTRUSTED CARE

We define entrusted care as health care in which major and minor decisions for treatment are made by a surrogate. Entrusted care can be *authorized* formally or informally by the patient to a family member, doctor, care manager, or combination of such persons. Or entrusted care might be *unauthorized*, as when a patient has a sudden brain trauma or stroke, has no immediate relatives, and has neglected to authorize anyone to make health care decisions for them.

Many degrees of entrusted care are possible, such as when a patient is dying and still has some input, but is too weak or scared or unsophisticated to formulate specific desires or make them known and acted upon. An instance of this is provided by my mother-in-law, who was informed by her doctor that her heart had stopped during her last dialysis. He told her that her chances for recovery were considerably less than had been previously thought. He then asked, "Do you want to be resuscitated should your heart stop during your next dialysis?" She was an uncomplicated person who perhaps did not fully understand the question or its gravity. Her response (to my dismay) was, "Do whatever you have to do." With those words, she entrusted her care and the difficult decisions to be made to her physician.

When patients place themselves by commission or omission into a situation of entrusted care, existing ethical criteria for decision making are (a) substituted judgment and (b) best interest. Decision making is supposed to occur with a clear understanding of what consequences would be most desirable from the patients' point of view.

Substituted Judgment

The principle of substituted judgment states that "in the absence of a written directive, a surrogate can come to the same decision the patient would if he were not incapacitated" (Robinson, 2001, p. 76). If the patient had detailed discussions with the surrogate regarding the use of specific treatments required by specific medical conditions, the principle of autonomy can still be upheld. Sometimes, though, even when another person has been designated by the patient to make health care decisions, the patient has not said anything definitive about his or her wishes or desired outcomes specific to the present health care situation. Or, family members may disagree about what was said, or that their loved one really meant what was said. (They may disagree with the patient's written advance directives as well.) In cases where family members disagree, no definitive decisions can be made and patients are usually kept on life support to prevent future litigation by family members who want to prolong life.

Best Interest Principle

The principle of best interest states that "when an incapacitated patient has not discussed his treatment preferences with the surrogate, the surrogate must apply general knowledge of the patient and the patient's values to treatment decisions" (Robinson, 2001, p. 76). Factors that should also be considered are prognosis, quality of life, consequences known to be important to the patient, and degree of suffering.

The chief problem with the best interest standard is that different and honorable persons will have varied and deeply vested interests about which prognosis matters, what will enhance or detract from quality of life, and how to assess the degree of suffering that will be experienced in the future as a result of decisions made in the present. Most older adults have several concurrent chronic illnesses with which they function well or marginally until some health change "puts them over the edge." In these cases, different specialists have different opinions about what is best for a patient. The case study of Ruth, below, is an example from my practice and it illustrates some shortcomings of the best interest principle.

Case Study: Decision Making—Alzheimer's Disease

Ruth was placed on my Alzheimer's unit because her advanced dementia made it impossible for her to live at home. After a few years in the nursing home, Ruth developed breast cancer which began fulminating. Her son did not want the mass to be treated, believing that any cancer treatment would be traumatic and futile in terms of Ruth's overall health trajectory. The medical director at the nursing home believed that conservative treatment was feasible and humane because the mass was causing a painful and open wound. The medical director consulted a surgeon who advocated excision of the mass, an oncologist who advocated mild chemotherapy, and a radiation specialist who believed radiation therapy would have the best results. Here were four different opinions from well-meaning individuals about the best interest of the patient. (We can see from this example that the best interest principle is highly subjective and fraught with power struggles about whose opinion prevails.) The family's preference for no treatment prevailed and the mass was suppurating and painful for more than a year before the patient died of complications from dementia.

An assumption of Comfort Care is that the human need for comfort is universal. Therefore, in the above case study, comfort might have been considered the consequence of highest importance for Ruth. If Comfort Care had been applied in the case study of Ruth, the family would have prioritized the comfort need arising from the fulminating open wound. Even in Ruth's advanced dementia, constant irritation from seepage, rubbing, intermittent infections, and bulky dressings caused anxiety and agitation. Perhaps conservative surgery would have set her back temporarily because of the anesthesia, tethers, and removal from her familiar environment, but her comfort would have been greatly enhanced over the long course of her primary disease of dementia. Additionally, the physical discomfort of a surgical procedure could have been treated by pain medications that do not cause additional confusion. Likewise, tethers such as a foley catheter and IV lines could have been removed in the immediate postoperative period. Psychospiritually, Ruth's comfort would have been enhanced because the anxiety of knowing something was terribly wrong with her breast would have been relieved. Environmentally, hospitalization would have caused temporary discomfort, but she could return as soon as possible to her familiar surroundings. Environmental discomforts also could have been relieved in the hospital by compensating with social comfort measures, such as the presence of beloved family members and nursing home staff. Had Ruth's son applied the framework of Comfort Care, he probably would have made a different decision based on the *overall* comfort needs of his mother—with plans for compensating for temporary comfort needs necessitated by a brief hospitalization.

Comfort Care as a Principle for Entrusted Care Decisions

I propose that Comfort Care be widely considered by many health care disciplines as a useful and more definitive model for decision making in cases of entrusted care. The advantages of Comfort Care over currently used ethical principles are several:

1.   Holistic Comfort Care reduces power struggles in entrusted care because the universal need for comfort (of the patient) provides a

strong basis for making health care decisions. The focus for decision making is on achieving the highest degree of holistic comfort for the patient. His or her comfort is the desired consequence and is achieved through deliberate choices toward that end. Comfort Care focuses decision makers away from their vested interests and beliefs, and toward the decision that will make the patient most comfortable *in a holistic sense.*

2.   The standard of Comfort Care is objective, because we can observe the consequences of health care choices that are made to enhance the patient's comfort. When physical sensations and mental perceptions are positive, patients appear relaxed and sleep well. They respond in peaceful ways to family members. Thus, the correctness of health care decisions is reinforced by observable indicators of the patient's comfort which, in many cases, occur immediately.

3.   The standard of Comfort Care is applied the same way across patients, accounting for each unique circumstance and set of known comfort preferences. The pattern is applied regardless of patients' ability or desire to participate in health care decisions. Comfort Care entails a *pattern* for making *individualized* decisions.

4.   Comfort Care is holistic because it entails physical, psychospirtual, sociocultural, and environmental comfort, and decisions are made on the basis of balancing all types of comfort to achieve a picture of the patients' total comfort level.

The next case study shows how conflicts among competing consequences were resolved using the framework of Comfort Care for ethical decision making.

Case Study: Decision Making—Living Will

Bill was my uncle, a kind and gentle man with a strong but unobtrusive faith. He had been in perfect health during his first 83 years, walking every day and living an idyllic life of rewarding self-employment in his own home. He then developed Parkinson's disease, noticeable first with mild dementia. At this time, he signed advance directives, stating that he did not want artificial feedings to prolong his death. He had a strong faith and wasn't afraid to die.

For the next 3 years, Bill lived at home, being cared for by his wife of 50 years. Bill's disease progressed, however, and he began falling several times a day. His confusion increased and his ability to perform activities of daily living decreased. His muscles were rigid and painful. His medications were increased, causing agitation, weakness, and catatonia and he had a small stroke. He couldn't swallow, which meant he couldn't take his Parkinson's medications. He could no longer express his treatment wishes.

We all knew that Bill did not want an artificial feeding tube, but without his medication to control symptoms of Parkinson's, he was so tremorous and tense that he appeared to be convulsing and was in severe pain and indignity. He had to be restrained in order to keep him from bouncing out of the bed. We, his loving and highly informed family, agreed to go against his previously expressed wishes for a quick and peaceful death because his physical condition prevented it. We authorized the placement of a feeding tube so he could receive his large doses of carbidopa/levodopa. However, this meant prolonging his death, because he would also receive nutrition. Bill was placed in a nursing home where he lay in a conscious and more comfortable state with feedings and medications administered in a continuous drip. He was unable to speak or participate in activities and he died in his sleep 6 months later.

This was a situation where competing consequences offered no clear, best choice. We felt badly about going against Bill's living will, but realized that none of us had known how uncomfortable and undignified his death would be without the feeding tube to administer his necessary medications. When the decision was made to make him physically more comfortable, I wanted to engage the support of hospice to gradually titrate down the feedings in honor of his wishes for a quicker death. His immediate family would not agree to that measure, but death in this case came mercifully anyway.

COMFORT CARE AT END OF LIFE

We are all familiar with the term Comfort Care as a choice among various advance directives. In some ways, this usage is congruent with the holistic sense of Comfort Care that I have been developing throughout this book. When practitioners and family members adhere to the patient's wish for "Comfort Care only," they can be guided by consideration of what interventions will or will not enhance the patient's comfort. Within this context, it is important to ascertain how the patient feels about artificial hydration and nutrition, as these two measures are often included under the category of "Comfort Care only" on printed forms for advance directives. The problem is that artificial hydration and nutrition often do not enhance the patient's comfort—they may be instituted to make the family or practitioner feel better about the care rendered in the shadows of impending death (Kolcaba & Fisher, 1996; Zerwekh, 1997).

Questions for Entrusted Caregivers at End of Life

The framework of holistic Comfort Care, as described in this book, helps nurses discuss with families important questions that arise when making end-of-life decisions for their loved ones. For example, nurses and families together can consider the following:

- Is intervention X a comfort measure?
- To whom does intervention X provide comfort?
- Whose comfort (patient, family, physician, nurse, administrator) is of primary concern?
- How can this family best be comforted so that the patient is more comfortable?
- Is there anyone I can call on to help with this decision?
- Have I communicated everything about the comfort needs and comfort measures that work to the next shift or the next visitors or the interdisciplinary team?

These questions can serve as important points of consideration in creating a patient-centered and integrated plan for comfort of the patient, family members, and staff (Kolcaba & Fisher, 1996, p. 70).

A Good Death

A "good death" has been described as being meaningful for all; it is a death that ends well for patient, health care workers, and family (Dozor & Addison, 1992). It is a time to say good-bye to each other and to sum up and find meaning in the patient's life. "Patients should die like they're being rocked to sleep in their mother's arms" (Dozor & Addison, 1992, p. 539). Conversely, a bad death has been described as an unfulfilling interaction in which feelings of being overwhelmed, helpless, guilty, or anxious were involved. Although these feelings were reported by medical residents working with dying patients (Dozor & Addison, 1992), the same feelings can be experienced by any or all participants during the dying process.

The framework of holistic Comfort Care is consistent with a good death because each participant in the process is proactive, thoughtful, and goal directed. Total comfort entails life review, resolved relationships, and hope for a peaceful release. Ideally, the goal of a comfortable death is articulated by the patient either in advance of, or during, the terminal events. The goal entails assumptions that specific comfort measures will ensure a natural and good death. When patients know that they will be comfortable in this holistic sense, they have no need for euthanasia.

Although the comfort framework provides a valuable and holistic structure for discussions, decision making, and action, Comfort Care has traditionally been viewed by patients, families, and interdisciplinary team members as a withdrawal of hope. The variability in the trajectory of critical illnesses contributes to this dilemma; it is not always possible to make definitive decisions about when to change the treatment goal from cure to care. As a guideline in difficult cases such as these, the framework for Comfort Care informally directs nurses and families to make judgments, not about whether or not death is inevitable, but rather about contributors to or detractors from patient comfort. These are meaningful and productive decisions in and of themselves, and anxiety about probable health outcomes can be relieved in favor of a focus on enhancing the patient's immediate state of comfort (Kolcaba & Fisher, 1996).

Hope

There is always a significant role for hope in these difficult situations. Health professionals want to and should offer hope to patients and families throughout the dying trajectory. What is to be hoped for, however, can be gently and gradually redefined as dying progresses.

Hope is characterized by the belief in a personal and better tomorrow and the expectation that a better tomorrow is truly possible and important. Hope is often oriented to immortality rather than mortal life (Hinds, 1984; Nowotny, 1989). When hope is defined in terms of the patient, the hopes of the physician (that he or she will be successful in restoring health) and family (that the patient will live) are secondary. Furthermore, creating misplaced hope is likely to create more discomforts for the patient (and eventually, the family) as the concrete inevitability of death increases. Thus, a patient's hope that death will be "good" is the realistic goal of holistic Comfort Care, whether instituted legally or informally. If the patient also hopes for a peaceful afterlife, that too is consistent with the reality of the dying patient (Kolcaba & Fisher, 1996).

When the treatment goal is changed from life prolongation to Comfort Care, even though the patient may be in an acute care setting, it is appropriate to adopt the hospice precept that all treatment decisions should be judged by whether they contribute to patient comfort (Orr, Paris, & Siegler, 1991). By design, the framework of Comfort Care is a positive, humanistic guide for caregiving, discussion, and decision making when the need for holistic Comfort Care is apparent.

This idea of Comfort Care is expanded from that in advance directives and includes all aspects of patient comfort, with considerations for family comfort. When nurses implement the framework in this expanded sense, Comfort Care strengthens the patient and family and is positively related to a peaceful death. The result is a family which is empowered to work through and assist in their loved one's death, and a patient who is allowed and encouraged to meet death with peace, dignity, and comfort (Kolcaba & Fisher, 1996). The third case study, below, highlights the role of hope in critical situations.

Case Study: Decision Making—Acute Care

Arthur was a 58-year-old man who had had a coronary artery bypass graft. One week later, he was readmitted to the intensive care unit with respiratory failure and massive gastrointestinal bleeding. He was placed on a ventilator, and other invasive lines were inserted. He needed multiple transfusions and medications to maintain his blood pressure. Two days later, Arthur developed severe abdominal pain, and a laparotomy revealed that his bowel was necrotic. He developed peritonitis. A colostomy was performed and the wound left open to facilitate healing.

After the colostomy, Arthur remained alert on the ventilator. Over the next 2 months, however, he developed liver failure, sepsis, and renal failure necessitating a shunt and daily dialysis. His primary physician communicated to the family that he was not ready to "give up hope," meaning that he thought Arthur could still get better. The family struggled with the physician's beliefs, plus the fact that before his original surgery, Arthur was healthy and vitally active. However, he wrote on a magic slate, "I am dying—no more."

Implementing the framework of Comfort Care assisted the family and nurses to address Arthur's acute comfort needs and gradually change the object of their hope. For example, the issue of physical comfort was complex because medication sufficient to bring relief from pain caused drowsiness, a state that

Arthur resented, especially during family visits. The family did not want to see Arthur in pain, so they reduced their visits with the idea that he would take more pain medication if he had fewer visitors. Gradually, they were made to see that Arthur wanted them to come, wanted to be alert for their visits, and that heightened physical pain during these visits was transcended by his social comfort when they were present. They all hoped for good visits in which Arthur was alert enough to participate, while medicated enough to be fairly comfortable.

Similarly, environmental needs were met when Arthur requested that the blinds be opened to let in light, even though the nurses had thought that the darkened room was more peaceful. Needs for privacy and quiet were also addressed. Arthur's communication needs were met with "yes-no" questions, the magic slate, and lip reading. At one point, he looked up at the nurse and mouthed, "I am going to die." The nurse nodded in agreement, for which Arthur expressed gratefulness and then asked the nurse to tell the family it was "okay." The mutual acknowledgment of imminent death was extremely comforting to nurses, Arthur, and his family.

Gradually the object of hope had changed from hope for a cure to hope for a "good death." Arthur requested that his family not be present when his life support was discontinued because it would be more difficult for them all. With specific circumstances agreed to by Arthur and his family, the ventilator was turned off and Arthur died peacefully, in the company of his favorite nurse. Arthur's wishes were fulfilled, and everyone's hope for a good death was proved realistic as it was brought into being (Kolcaba & Fisher, 1996).

VIRTUE ETHICS OF CARE AND COMPASSION

Caring about someone can involve desire or romantic interest, but philosopher Lawrence Blum would say that this type of caring, while good, is not morally significant because it is not a virtue (1992, p. 125). Rather, romantic caring is an emotion which usually does not include the intellectual component of morality, at least in Western culture. Nurses, however, are expected to care about their patients and want what is good for them. In this way, caring is distinct from the simple recognition of a duty toward patients, though of course caring can coexist with more purely intellectual and benevolent states of mind. At times, caring may involve undertaking an unpleasant but helpful task, because we care for the other person's good.

Care also involves an openness or responsiveness toward the other. We cannot assume that we know what the other's good consists of, but we should be guided by the other's own reality. Thus, the reality of what actions, alone or combined, *actually* enhance each patient's comfort is a guide to decision making. Actual comfort is observed in the demeanor, behaviors, or words of the patient. We are not left to assume we know best, because the patient lets us know one way or another.

It is surprising to me that care and compassion for patients are not inherent in nursing's codes of ethics (Appendixes G and H), given that these qualities (ethical virtues) are generally considered to be aspects of common morality for health care providers. The writers of the codes omitted virtues, though, and the documents sound dry and intellectual as a result. Through omission, are the nurse writers implying that virtuous practice is supererogatory? Are caring and compassion above the call of duty? I should hope not, for the sake of our patients and the discipline.

Many of the comfort measures that nurses and other health care providers routinely offer to their patients fall under the category of professional obligations. Some comfort measures that used to be professional obligations, however, like back rubs, now might be considered "above and beyond the call of duty" by practitioners and/or administrators, especially with stressful patient assignments. Certainly, nurses need time and encouragement to perform such comfort measures, and extra comfort measures are usually the first ones cut when staffing is short. It is these types of comfort measures, however, that are recalled when patients think back on special nurses and others who excelled in helping family members or themselves through difficult health care situations. When talking with student nurses, I refer to these especially virtuous nurses as *memorable.*

MEMORABLE NURSES

When I introduce Comfort Care to my students, I begin by asking who in the group has been hospitalized or has had a close family member hospitalized for a serious illness or injury. Usually, several students raise their hands. Then I ask whether any of them remember the nurses during this stressful time. Only a few hands are left, and I ask those students to tell their stories. Sometimes I hear stories of nurses who were impatient or rough (Nurse Ratchet types are memorable, too) but there are always a few stories about very special, kind, thoughtful nurses. I ask the students to give some specific examples of what those nurses did that made them memorable. The stories are much like the model case in chapter 5 and from which the above quote was taken. That is, fondly remembered nurses are those who comforted their patients and family members. Memorable nurses took time to explain procedures, hold their patients' hands, reassure, encourage, give massages, straighten rooms, bring in special food, keep promises, etc. While the nurses also were competent, the patients or families especially remembered the kindnesses, compassion, and individualized care that these nurses gave. Not one student ever mentioned that a nurse was memorable because of his or her command of technology! (Although an incompetent nurse will surely bring about patient discomfort.)

Then I ask the students whether they hope to be memorable nurses in the positive sense. I tell them that the Theory of Comfort gives them a pattern for being this kind of nurse. Moreover, Comfort Care is efficient, individualized, and holistic—it is what patients want from their nurses. I describe how they, as practicing nurses, can save time by asking patients about their comfort needs, "clicking off" the four contexts of comfort in an informal assessment process. That is, is this patient comfortable: physically, psychospiritually, socioculturally, and environmentally? When comfort needs are identified, many of them can be addressed in one patient encounter, in actions so smooth and seamless that patients don't realize they have been comforted. Moreover, after the nurse leaves the room, the patient is usually fully satisfied and doesn't put the call light on any time soon. Such is the beauty and simplicity of Comfort Care.

When we practice Comfort Care, we intuit that the four categories of comfort needs are interrelated and that total comfort is more than the sum of its parts. For example, acute pain causes anxiety that can lead to immobility, dysfunction, and feelings of helplessness. On the other hand, a back rub addresses many needs for comfort, such as loneliness, tension, anxiety, and insomnia, and has many positive effects on patients beyond what one would expect from a single intervention. Also, while nurses usually spend more time with patients than other practitioners, any discipline can foster "memorable" care providers.

MUSINGS ON COMFORT QUOTE (CHAPTER 8)

> I made a finer end, and he went away as if he had been any Christian child. He parted just between twelve and one, for after I saw him fumble with the sheets, and play with

flowers, and smile upon his fingers' end, I knew there was but one way. . . . "How now, Sir John! What, man, be of good cheer." So he cried out, "God, God, God!" three or four times. Now I, to comfort him, bid him he should not think of God; I hoped there was no need to trouble himself with any such thought yet. So he bade me lay more clothes on his feet; I put my hand into the bed and felt them, and they were as cold as any stone.
—William Shakespeare (1598), *King Henry the Fifth*, Act 2, Scene 3 (Death scene of Falstaff as told by Hostess Quigley)

In this quote, Hostess Quigley describes the care she gave Falstaff that went beyond her duties as a hotel clerk. Her acts of kindness displayed the virtue of compassion.

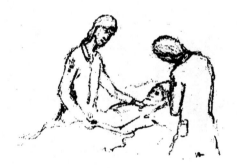

CHAPTER 9

Mission Updated

First and foremost, human beings—worldwide—want to be
comforted and kept safe by nursing care.
—M. Mallison, Editor, *American Journal
of Nursing*, 1990, p. 15

We labour soon, we labour late to feed the titled knave, man;
And ah the comfort we're to get, is that beyond the grave, man.
—Robert Burns, Scottish poet (1838), *The Tree of Liberty*

In chapter 7, I described comfort studies in which groups that received specific comfort measures (interventions or treatments) demonstrated statistically significant differences in comfort over time,
compared to a control group. In addition, some of the studies measured
relationships between comfort and designated health seeking behaviors
(HSBs) such as the two urinary incontinence studies (Dowd, Kolcaba, &
Steiner, 2000; Dowd, Kolcaba, & Steiner, 2002). Since that time, a new
variable for the Theory of Comfort has been added and further premises
have been developed. This chapter discusses why and how the new

variable, *Institutional Integrity* (InI)[1], was added to the theoretical model. Conceptual and operational definitions of this variable are presented. This chapter also contains my thoughts about institutional outcomes, indicators of nurse productivity, and current initiatives in professional nursing.

THEORY OF COMFORT EVOLVES
FOR OUTCOMES RESEARCH

Background

The emphasis on hospital outcomes in the late 20th century came as a result of managed care, which represented a sea change in the way health care was delivered. Before managed care, physicians had unlimited freedom to order diagnostic tests, perform procedures, decide on length of hospital stay, and prescribe medications. Government-run programs, such as Medicaid and Medicare, reimbursed physicians and/ or diagnostic departments and/or hospitals for every service performed and every hospital day. Neither government nor private insurance companies utilized oversight capabilities or regulations to keep health care costs down or to prevent illness. Under this "fee-for-service" system, prevalent up through the mid-1980s, the practice of medicine was lucrative and hospitals were plentiful and profitable.

Eventually, the economic resources of the government and private insurance companies were severely stressed by uncontrolled health care costs. Economists urged more oversight to control expenses and reduce the percent of the gross national product spent on health care. Early discharges, based on diagnostic related groups (DRGs), became the norm but with minimal support for families caring for their sick loved ones at home. While the development and cost of new pharmaceuticals and technology continued unabated, hospitals, home health services, and nursing homes received less and less money for services provided. Health promotion and disease prevention remained on the back burner. By the early 1990s, public and private health care providers were in financial crisis.

---

[1]InI is used to abbreviate Institutional Integrity, instead of II. This format represents a slight deviation from APA format and is done because II is naturally interpreted as "two." Readers who miss the first usage of InI for Institutional Integrity will, at least, know that they need to find out what it means instead of misreading it.

In the mid-1990s, competition increased among hospitals because, to stay afloat, it was necessary to fill beds with patients well covered by insurance. Most people below age 65 were insured through their employers and only if they worked full time in large businesses. Employers chose insurance plans for their employees. In turn, insurance companies began deciding which hospital their enrollees would use. Therefore, hospital administrators had to demonstrate to insurers that their patients had better outcomes than the hospital down the road. Also, to cut costs, preventive medicine began to be encouraged by insurers and community-based nurses reemphasized their health promotion activities. Managed care systems took on oversight responsibilities and eventually made treatment decisions based in large part on economics.

Because most physicians billed patients separately for their services, their fees were not immediately or drastically jeopardized by managed care. Nurses, however, were salaried by hospitals for providing a wide range of unspecified services, and immediately became vulnerable to the budgetary constraints of their employers. Then and now, professional nurse staffing was viewed as a large, but supposedly flexible, percent of institutional budgeting. Thus, nursing staff was cut in administrators' efforts to keep their institutions financially viable.

By 2001, with bare-bones hospital staffing, nurses no longer had time to assess and address comfort needs in their patients. They ran from one acutely ill patient to another, reacting to emergency situations, quickly discharging patients who were still sick or weak, and almost immediately admitting new and sicker patients, all of which generated a tremendous amount of paperwork and stress for staff nurses. Nurses were fearful of making errors or failing to notice untoward symptoms in their very sick patients because they were busy elsewhere. Mandatory overtime was imposed in lieu of continuous adequate staffing. The practice of hospital nursing became less autonomous and less professional. For these reasons, many nurses left nursing or moved to more professional environments such as teaching or private business.

Advocacy groups for nurses began looking at institutional outcomes in efforts to balance standards of good care with cost saving measures. At first, analysts looked at negative outcomes such as patient mortality, infection rates, bedsores, errors, length of stay, and hospital readmissions. Report cards on these outcomes and others were published and sometimes discredited by hospitals that did poorly. Those hospitals then refused to release further data. The "report card" system, created to help consumers and managed care groups make comparisons among competing institutions, failed because of poor cooperation among hospitals. Early studies done by these groups and other researchers, however, began to point out relationships between low professional nurse staffing and increased incidence of negative outcomes.

The American Nurses Association measured and compared three categories of indicators: structure, process, and patient outcomes, sometimes correlating them with each other. For example, data about nurse-patient ratios (structure) in different institutions were compared with their rates of nosocomial infection (outcome). These data conclusively demonstrated that higher staffing levels of professional nurses resulted in a decrease in negative outcomes such as urinary tract infection, pneumonia, shock, upper gastrointestinal bleeding, and increased length of stay (Buerhaus & Needleman, 2000; Foley, 2001; HRSA, 2001; Saltus, 2001). (These data were from medical patients.)

These data were important for nursing because they demonstrated empirically that patients did much better as professional nurse staffing increased. In this era of competition, hospitals did better in the business world when their patients did better. The outcomes that were measured, though, were negative. Another example was an important outcome measure for surgical patients. It was called "failure to rescue," defined as the death rate among patients with sepsis, pneumonia, shock, upper gastrointestinal bleeding, or deep vein thrombosis (HRSA, 2001).

We have known for a long time that hospitals are dangerous places, and the above reports bear this out. But patients who must be hospitalized want and need more than to be "rescued" from hospital acquired infections, hemorrhage, shock, or errors in medications or treatments. They want and need to be cared for, not by a family member, but by a professional nurse. They want and need reassurance, information, touch, and personalized care. In short, in today's high-tech health care arena they want *comfort* more than ever (Kolcaba, 2000). If the profession of nursing is to remain valued by patients, we must deliver what patients want and expect from their nurses.

Retroduction

The health care climate described above made me realize that Comfort Theory had to address the deteriorating realities for professional nursing specifically, and for patient care in general. One way to do this would be through research to demonstrate the value of holistic patient care, conditional on adequate staffing and a professional working environment. A new concept was needed in the Theory of Comfort that would guide thinking and research along these lines.

Retroduction is a form of reasoning that originates ideas. It is useful for selecting and naming phenomena that can be developed further and tested. This type of reasoning is applied in fields in which there are few available theories (Bishop, 1998). Outcomes research is a field of inquiry that has emerged in nursing and other disciplines in response to managed care. It utilizes large databases from hospital populations or regional populations, for a 1- or 5-year period (for example). Selected patient interventions and/or outcomes are measured through questionnaires and chart review and those variables are then related to types of nursing, staffing levels, organizational structures, or financial goals.

As discussed earlier, Murray's 20th century framework could not account for 21st century emphasis on institutional outcomes. Therefore, InI was added to the Mid-Range Theory of Comfort at the end of line 4, Figure 9.1. InI is defined conceptually as "the quality or state of health care organizations being complete, whole, sound, upright, professional, and ethical providers of health care" (Kolcaba, 2001, p. 89).

One goal for adapting the Theory of Comfort was to demonstrate that institutions with higher nurse staffing, professional atmospheres, and patient-oriented value systems were more likely to reach their specific financial and health-related goals. If this positive relationship were revealed in the data, results would get the attention and support from hospital and agency administrators for truly professional environments in which nurses and team members could provide the best care they knew how to provide. Therefore, three propositions were added to the list of original Comfort Theory propositions and are listed below. They are numbered 7, 8, and 9. The complete list of theoretical propositions is given in Figure 9.1.

7. When patients engage in HSBs as result of being strengthened by comfort care, nurses and patients are more satisfied with health care and patients demonstrate better health-related (diagnosis specific) outcomes.
8. A professional working environment produces better patient and institutional outcomes.
9. When patients and nurses are satisfied with health care in a specific institution, public acknowledgment about the institution's commitment to health in the United States will contribute

Line 4

Health + Nursing + Intervening → **Enhanced** → Health → Institutional
Care   Interventions   Variables   **Comfort**   Seeking   Integrity
Needs   Behaviors

Propositions in Adapted Theory of Comfort

1. Nurses identify patients' and/or families' comfort needs that have not been met by existing support systems.
2. Nurses design interventions to address those needs.
3. Intervening variables are taken into account in designing the interventions and determining whether they have probability for success.
4. If the intervention is effective, and delivered in a caring manner, the immediate outcome of enhanced comfort is attained and the intervention is a comfort measure. Comfort Care entails all of these components.
5. Patients and nurses agree upon desirable and realistic health seeking behaviors (HSBs).
6. If enhanced comfort is achieved, patients are strengthened to engage in HSBs which further enhances comfort.
7. When patients engage in HSBs as result of being strengthened by Comfort Care, nurses and patients are more satisfied with health care and demonstrate better health related (diagnosis specific) outcomes.
8. A professional working environment produces better patient and institutional outcomes.
9. When patients and nurses are satisfied with health care in a specific institution, public acknowledgment about the institutions' commitment to health in the United States will contribute to institutions remaining viable and flourishing.

FIGURE 9.1   Theoretical framework for Comfort Care related to institutional integrity.

Figure 9.1 adapted with permission from Kolcaba, K. (2001). Evolution of the mid-range theory of comfort for outcomes research. *Nursing Outlook, 49*(2), 86–92.

to institutions remaining viable and flourishing (see discussion about magnet designation later in this chapter).

Operationalizing Institutional Integrity

Although outcomes research has thus far focused on negative outcomes, InI is generally a desired outcome and can be measured (operationalized) in a variety of positive ways. The first and most readily available data are from surveys about *patient and/or family satisfaction.* This is information that most hospitals and agencies are already collecting for competitive purposes. A second example of InI is *successful discharges,* which can be operationalized as the number of patients who avoid readmission to the hospital within 6 months for problems related to the condition(s) causing the original hospitalization. A third example of InI is *length of stay* (LOS). Data about LOS are readily available in institutional data banks. A fourth example of InI is *financial stability* of hospitals or agencies. Obviously, financial data can be gathered only through the cooperation of each institution.

Currently, I am developing ways in which to test the last part of the theory; that is, demonstrating that positive relationships exist between patients' comfort in an institutional setting, their engagement in health seeking behaviors, and the extent of their satisfaction with care as surveyed after discharge. Comfort Theory postulates that an intentional emphasis on and support for Comfort Care by an institution will be "rewarded" by increased satisfaction *because* persons are healed, strengthened, and motivated to be engaged more fully in HSBs. If this theory stands up to testing, institutions will have more evidence that Comfort Care matters, not only for recipients of care, but for the viability of those institutions.

Note that institutional commitments to Comfort Care are extremely important for patient comfort because providing a full range of Comfort Care may be difficult in stressful health care climates. Emphasis on professional working environments, patient-oriented value systems, and changes in ways that we currently measure nurse productivity, can make intentional Comfort Care valued once again.

NURSING-SENSITIVE OUTCOMES

Patient outcomes have emerged as essential measures of health care quality in managed care systems. Although a number of patient outcome measures are now available, there has been minimal emphasis on the identification and measurement of positive outcomes for the evaluation of nursing interventions. These outcomes are directly related to nursing interventions and, to support our profession, are nursing sensitive. That is, patient outcomes are those that are influenced most by the practice of nursing (Johnson & Maas, 1999).

Outcome measurement is an essential component of quality evaluation and effectiveness research. As stated previously, to facilitate continual quality improvement, information about patient outcomes should identify not only negative outcomes but also those that are marginal, adequate, or superior (Johnson & Maas, 1999). A schema for outcomes research that helps clarify different types of outcomes is presented in the two concentric circles illustrated in Figure 9.2. The inner circle, or core, contains global and multidisciplinary patient outcomes such as health status and satisfaction. The outer circle contains three types of intermediate outcomes: diagnosis specific, discipline specific, and system specific.

The outcome of patient comfort is a good example of a positive, discipline specific outcome because it reflects the practice and standards in nursing and it is capable of measuring the effectiveness of comfort

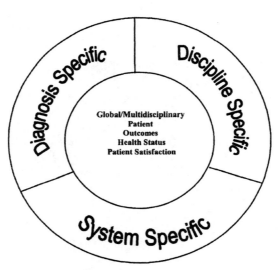

FIGURE 9.2   Categories of outcomes.

Used by permission: Johnson, M., & Maas, M. (1999). Nursing-sensitive patient outcomes. In E. Cohen & V. DeBack (Eds.), *The outcomes mandate* (p. 39). St. Louis: Mosby.

measures with individuals and aggregates. This intermediate, discipline specific outcome also influences the health and satisfaction of patients.

NEED FOR STANDARDIZED NURSING-SENSITIVE OUTCOME MEASURES

In addition to identifying discipline-specific patient outcome measures for nursing, it is equally important that these measures be standardized and validated. If the nursing profession is to become a full participant in clinical evaluation, it is essential that patient outcomes influenced by nursing care be measured in conjunction with outcomes important to other disciplines and to the patient. Furthermore, participation in clinical evaluation and policy making requires that standardized nursing data be included in integrated, computerized, clinical informational systems (Johnson & Maas, 1999).

Several uniform data sets have been developed for the U.S. health care delivery system, such as the Uniform Hospital Discharge Data Set (Health Information Policy Council, 1985), the Uniform Ambulatory Medical Care Minimum Data Set (National Committee on Vital and Health Statistics, 1981), and the Long Term Care Minimum Data Set (National Committee on Vital and Health Statistics, 1980). Although many of these data sets provide valuable information about systems and organizations, they do not always determine nursing care effectiveness. When researchers fail to investigate nursing care effectiveness, decision making and policy development that are crucial to the viability of nursing in general are made without specific nursing data. This is true for any auxiliary health care discipline as well.

I have been encouraged to note that patient comfort is cited as an outcome on several classification schemes such as the one compiled by Jennings, Staggers, and Brosch (1999), a report card template proposed by the American Nurses Association (ANA; Derman & Huber, 1999), and the Iowa Project Nursing Outcomes Classification (NOC) system (Nursing Outcomes Classification, 2000, p. 173). I believe that the NOC system offers the most promise for a schema of positive outcomes that can and is being applied across many nursing specialties to measure the effectiveness of nursing interventions in those specialties. The NOC system has its corresponding Nursing Intervention Classification (NIC) system to measure the effectiveness of common nursing interventions for achieving selected similarly classified outcomes.

Note that any nurse can measure comfort in patients and any nurse can request that his or her unit selects comfort as an outcome measurement in small or large research projects. If we think that patient comfort matters, and seek a more professional environment in which to effect patient comfort, we need to *show* that it matters. In addition, we need to show that our institutions can benefit by our commitment (and theirs) to Comfort Care.

I was pleased that the American Nurses Credentialing Center is encouraging health care organizations to develop and implement models and practices to make institutions more attractive for nurses. Such facilities that have developed best practices can now be granted the "magnet" designation (American Nurses Association, 2001). Outcomes research has demonstrated that magnet facilities consistently have nurse retention that is twice as long as that in non-magnet facilities. More importantly, patients have fewer negative outcomes; shorter lengths of stay, and increased satisfaction with their health care services (American Nurses Association, 2001). My hope is that Comfort Care will become one of those models for best practices and that the obvious related, positive outcome of increased patient comfort will be a valued goal for magnet institutions. For this to happen, nurses must document comfort as an outcome of holistic care in a seamless flow of practice and outcome measurement (Buerhaus & Norman, 2001).

CLINICAL PRACTICE GUIDELINES
FOR PAIN AND COMFORT

The American Society of Perianesthesia Nurses (ASPAN) is in the process of preparing their "Clinical Practice Guidelines for Pain and Comfort." That proactive group of nurses believe, and I concur, that these guidelines will be the first in any nursing specialty to address both phenomena close to the hearts of our patients: pain and comfort. I was privileged to present what I knew about patient comfort to their consensus conference held in January 2002. The purpose of the consensus conference was to obtain feedback from perianesthesia nurses from around the country about what should be included in the practice guidelines.

Kicking off the conference were experts germane to the consensus process and to pain and comfort. The presenters gave background about (a) requirements for practice guidelines in general, (b) postsurgical pain, (c) comfort, and (d) future directions for practice guidelines from the perspective of the Joint Commission for Hospital Accreditation. I learned a lot from these experts and gained some new insights when feedback about my presentations was given.

A phrase from the cofounder of the American Society of Pain Management Nurses, Chris Pasero, stuck in my mind. She said, "This is the decade for pain management." Her prognosis was indeed welcomed by the perianesthesia nurses and was a long time coming. Later I stated that perhaps the next decade would be the decade for comfort management! It was certainly the intent of ASPAN to thrust comfort into nurses' awareness sooner than 2010, but this was only one nursing specialty. We all know that paradigm shifts, such as talking about and ministering to holistic comfort as well as pain, take considerable time to be accepted, translated into practice, and included in mandates from accrediting bodies such as the Joint Commission. Ten years, therefore, seems just about right for a real paradigm shift to comfort in health care to occur. (I'll keep my fingers not crossed, but busy at the keyboard in the meantime!)

Comfort

My presentation began with the definition of holistic comfort—which is in your glossary and elsewhere in this book. Reiterating, comfort is the immediate experience of being strengthened by having needs for Relief, Ease, and Transcendence met in four contexts (physical, psychospiritual, sociocultural, and environmental). As you recall, this definition arose with the taxonomic structure (TS) of comfort (Figure 1.2) and was later applied through the Theory of Comfort. I also explained to the audience how cells in the TS were attributes of comfort. Naturally, the nurses also heard Comfort Theory, as well as its major propositions (Figure 9.1). The following assumptions, expanded from the assumptions of whole-person holism in chapter 4, were included in the presentation:

- Comfort is a desirable, strengthening, holistic outcome that is germane to the discipline of nursing and health care.
- Human beings strive to meet, or to have met, their basic comfort needs. It is an active endeavor.
- The effects of comfort measures are perceived with six senses (touch, smell, taste, hearing, seeing, proprioception).
- Comfort is individualistic and more than the absence of pain.

Pain

When guidelines are constructed for nursing specialties, a glossary of terms is a good idea to ensure that all users of the guidelines are on the same page. Therefore, many of the terms in this book's glossary were put into a perianesthesia glossary, and some new ones were developed for the specialty.The definition of pain that I used is a multidimensional discomfort including sensory, cognitive, and affective components (Melzak & Wall, 1982).

Focal Pain

For the conference, I coined the term "focal pain" to designate a specific, severe, expected, and relatively localized pain associated with a surgical procedure. I found the term to be useful in discussions about the relationship between pain and comfort, because there are different types of pain. Focal pain is the focus of postoperative pain management, however, and, if not managed, focal pain is a significant detractor from comfort. For other specialties, focal pain would be associated with contractions during labor and delivery, or medical problems such as cancer, trauma, migraine headaches, or vertebral collapse. To conform to the idea of focal pain, the pain is acute, and (hopefully) time-limited. Focal pain can also be called a severe discomfort.

The Relationship Between Comfort and Pain

The TS is useful for describing the relationship between comfort and focal pain. Focal pain is located in the TS cell "physical relief" and, when not relieved, can be the major detractor from holistic comfort. (Remember that there can be other discomforts in this cell such as nausea, vomiting, constipation, hunger for food or air, thirst, electrolyte imbalance, and other physiological problems of which the patient may or may not be aware.) Picturing this arrangement between pain and comfort, it is clear that comfort is an umbrella term under which effective pain management is a significant part. Congruent with Melzak's definition above, focal pain also has affective, cognitive, and sensory components. But pain management isn't the only aspect of comfort (there are 11 other cells as well as other possible candidates for physical relief). The relationship between pain relief and comfort is much more complex.

Pain Intensifiers

Dr. Paul Brand (Yancey & Brand, 1997) describes how he felt during his own hospitalization.

> Despite my medical background I felt helpless, inadequate, and passive. I had the overwhelming impression of being reduced to a cog in a machine, and a malfunctioning cog at that. Every sound filtering in from the hallway somehow related to my predicament. A rolling cart—they must be coming for me. A groan from the hallway—Oh no, they've found something. (1997, pp. 262–263)

Brandt coined the phrase "pain intensifiers," which he defined as responses that heighten the perception of pain within the conscious mind (p. 262). He describes how intensifiers such as anxiety, fear, anger, guilt, loneliness, and helplessness may have more impact on the overall experience of (focal) pain than any prescription drug available. To fulfill our dual mission of effective pain management and enhancement of comfort, nurses must determine what stimuli cause or might cause these individualistic negative responses that make pain worse, and then intervene appropriately.

The idea of pain intensifiers illustrates how important it is for nurses to attend to patients' holistic comfort: this is a way to achieve the most effective and efficient management of focal pain. Pain and comfort are intimately linked: as comfort is enhanced in other cells of the TS, focal pain diminishes. The three types of comfort measures (interventions) discussed in chapter 5 can all be utilized as adjuncts to opioids and other analgesics in treating focal pain. Treating anxiety, before it reaches panic levels, may be the *best* care plan for pain management because less opioids will be required than would be expected for a particular type of focal pain (Yancey & Brand, 1997).

Recommendations for Clinical Practice Guidelines for Pain and Comfort

Based on the input of more than 100 nurses reaching consensus about pain and comfort management, the following recommendations can be made:

1. When taking medical histories, ask about predispositions/risk factors for heightened focal pain, such as high anxiety, previous experiences with pain, chronic discomforts, etc.

2. Confusion produces anxiety, so those who are prone to post-procedure confusion, or those who are confused for other reasons, will need all sensory aides in place (dentures, eye glasses, hearing aids, canes or walkers). When possible, for these patients, encourage regional blocks instead of general anesthesia.
3. Advocate for the most suitable anesthetic/pain management strategies for each specific patient.
4. Ask patients (and or families) about existing detractors from comfort and identify and treat current pain intensifiers.
5. Ask about comfort measures that have worked for patients previously, and "pass it on" to provide personalized continuity of care. This also increases patients' confidence.
6. Provide thorough education about focal pain to be expected for a specific condition or procedure, and the best options for managing it, including complementary therapies. When possible, encourage patients to choose among options.
7. Determine post-procedure comfort and pain management goals prior to the procedure. For pathological pain in cases like cancer, determine comfort and pain management goals. For example, comfort sufficient for rest or for function? Comfort goals will change with circumstances.
8. After comfort and pain management strategies have been instituted, practitioners must ask the right questions, and ask them frequently. For example, it may be more positive and less frightening to be asked, "How is your comfort?" and "How is your pain control?" rather than being asked to rate one's pain from 1–10, with 10 being as bad as it can possibly be. ("You mean my pain could get worse?")
9. Establish institutional guidelines for frequency of assessment and documentation.
10. Document each and every pain and comfort assessment, indicating how previously established goals are being met and which interventions are effective.

Assessment, Measurement, and Documentation

For research, we have found that comfort questionnaires provide the most reliable data. Comfort questionnaires can vary in length or content depending on the patient population. Perianesthesia nurses tell me that patients can't cope with a lot of questions postoperatively, however, and the nurses prefer to ask one or two simple questions such as those above in recommendation number 8. Another option is the visual analog scale which our hospice patients find easy to understand, but may be inappropriate with postoperative patients because of vision difficulties. Regardless of institutional choices, the important things are to a) ask frequently about focal pain and comfort, b) document patients' responses consistently, and c) determine which interventions have been effective.

NURSE PRODUCTIVITY

Just a note about the way "bean counters" measure nurse productivity. Currently, the *number* of patients to which a nurse is assigned on any given day (perhaps accounting for patient acuity) is usually considered that nurse's productivity. It can be measured for an individual nurse, a unit, or an institution. Supposedly, nurse productivity is analogous to factory worker productivity. In a factory, the number of widgets a worker finishes in one day is the measure of his or her productivity. If we think about it, though, the number and kind of patients in a nursing assignment is actually analogous to the *raw material* brought into a factory. The finished widget, without defects, is the desired *factory outcome* and the measure of factory worker productivity. Likewise, *desired patient outcomes* such as comfort, quick healing, early ambulation, return to previous function, adherence to a rehabilitation plan (without a quick readmission for the same medical problem), and even patient satisfaction *should be* the measures of productivity in a given hospital or agency. According to Comfort Theory, these desired positive outcomes can come about more efficiently and completely if patients' holistic comfort needs are addressed. Nurses need institutional support and reinforcement for delivering Comfort Care in order to achieve these desirable disease-related goals.

An institutional commitment to Comfort Care assures that nurse staffing is sufficient and the environment positive. Only then can nurses implement the three classic types of Comfort Measures or interventions: technical comfort measures, coaching, and comfort food for the soul (described in detail in chapter 5). Comfort Care embodies the art and science of nursing, and in showing the value of patient comfort, we also highlight the high level of skill and caring that bring about holistic comfort. Comfort Theory claims that, when nurses have time and support to practice Comfort Care, their patients will have better outcomes, which is the *actual* measure of nurse productivity and InI. The institution wins in another way as well. Nurse satisfaction will increase while nurse turnover and absenteeism will decrease.

INNOVATIVE MODELS OF COMFORT CARE UTILIZING INSTITUTIONAL INTEGRITY

1. Hospice Care

The purpose of this pilot study was to determine whether a simple intervention like hand massage, given twice a week by trained nurse researchers, could enhance holistic comfort of persons who are faced with a terminal diagnosis. If the immediate outcome of comfort was enhanced, we hypothesized that patients would also experience a peaceful death, a health seeking behavior (Kolcaba, 1994).

Comfort Care is a natural fit with hospice nursing because it includes spiritual care in its theoretical base. Comfort is also an important goal for care as stated in Standards for Hospice Care (American Nurses Association, 1991, 1994; National Hospice Organization, 1994). Following the Comfort Care framework (Figure 9.3), we identified the known comfort needs of hospice patients that our team became familiar with in earlier work and from reviewing the literature. We also talked with hospice nurses, chaplains, physicians, and social workers. We plotted the comfort needs on a comfort grid (taxonomic structure [TS]) and designed our intervention to address as many needs as possible.

This hand massage intervention was chosen because it was easy to teach and to learn. When data collection was finished, professional and/or nonprofessional caregivers were shown how to do the massage and were given an instruction pamphlet for reinforcement of the protocol. Because this seemed to be a very powerful intervention for "connecting" the caregiver and care recipient, we hoped that it would be integrated into the daily routines of family members and/or professional caregivers.

Our research team was trained to perform the massage by a licensed massage therapist on our faculty. Important components of the massage that she included were (a) the approach to the patient and family, (b) preparing the environment, (c) explaining the procedure, (d) establishing trust and rapport, and (e) timing. These factors were included as

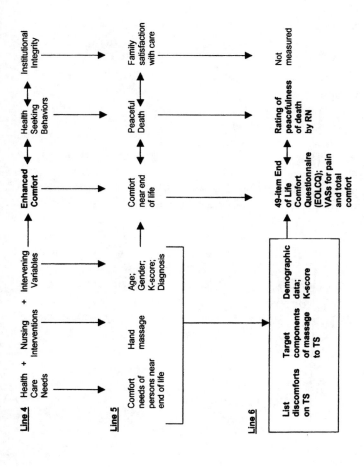

FIGURE 9.3 Theoretical framework for study of hand massage to enhance comfort and peacefulness of death in persons near end of life.

Note: Boldface indicates operational variables measured in this study (Dowd, Kolcaba, & Steiner, 2000).

integral parts of the written protocol that we developed because they helped to assure that the intervention covered the content domain of comfort, as designated by our comfort grid. The written protocol was necessary so that everyone on our research team would approach the patient and family the same way and perform the actual massage with the same technique.

We obtained our sample from two hospice agencies in northeast Ohio and one in New York State, by attending team conferences, identifying possible patients who met our inclusion criteria, contacting those persons, and obtaining permission to come to their homes to begin the study. Once in their homes, we explained the study in more detail and, if they still wanted to participate, the patients signed an informed consent. After signing the informed consent, patients picked an envelope with their group assignment written inside (Treatment or Comparison). Thus we accomplished random assignment to groups, and patients saw that there was no bias about which group they were in.

Demographic data plus a Karnofsky score (Appendix E), which was an observed functional level (Karnofsky & Burchenal, 1949), provided us with potential covariates (intervening variables) for data analysis. We used the End of Life Comfort Instruments developed and pilot tested earlier (Novak, Kolcaba, Steiner, & Dowd, 2001) to measure change in comfort over time after patients received the intervention twice a week for 3 consecutive weeks (Appendix F). This 49-item questionnaire was designed to cover the content domain of comfort, as guided by the TS. Each item has six possible responses; 1 = strongly disagree, through 6 = strongly agree. So, if a patient felt "sort of" relaxed (s)he picked number 4 as the response and if the patient was breathing easily, (s)he picked number 1 as the response. Some patients were able to work on the questionnaires independently, while others preferred that we read the questions to them. In that case, we provided them with 5 × 8 cards with the numbers written out and the anchors, strongly disagree and strongly agree, written above 1 and 6 respectively. Participants would hold the card and answer each question as spontaneously as possible.

Each patient's total comfort score was the sum of all the responses and higher scores indicated higher comfort. This is the format for all of the comfort questionnaires that we have developed so far, and in our instrumentation study of how well the questionnaire performed, 93 hospice patients did not express difficulties answering 49 questions (Novak et al., 2001). Other nurse researchers, however, thought the questionnaire was too long for patients near the end of life. So, a different group of 14 experts in hospice care rated the items for priority to include in a shortened instrument. They sent the results to me, and I mapped those priority items on a TS, adjusting some of the items for balance so the whole content domain of comfort was covered evenly. Our team decided to use the bolded items (shown in Appendix F), only when patients could not complete the full questionnaire.

We also used two visual analog scales to measure Total Comfort and Pain. If the participants died before the end of the study, the extent of peacefulness of death, our health seeking behavior, was assessed by the primary nurse on a vertical line, with 1 being at one end and 5 being at the other end. We collected data from each participant at the beginning of the study, once during the second week, and at the end of the study. In the treatment group, data were collected before the hand massage took place so patients could remain relaxed after the intervention. These patients received hand massage twice a week for 3 weeks.

Because this was a pilot study, subsequent to procuring larger funding, we did not investigate relationships between enhanced comfort, peaceful death, and desirable institutional outcomes such as family satisfaction with care. Rather we felt that we first needed to obtain empirical evidence of the benefits of hand massage for enhancing comfort and peacefulness of death. If pilot data (quantitative and qualitative) support the intervention's relationship to enhanced comfort and a peaceful death, we will include the testing of the larger theory by adding InI variables and enrolling several agencies. Those InI variables will be ones in which our participating hospice agencies are interested, such as family satisfaction with care and/or a cost-benefit analysis of the intervention.

2. Acute Care for Elders (ACE)

ACE is a model of care for older adults in acute care hospitals that arose from a collaborative effort in northeast Ohio between geriatricians, nurses, social workers, and hospital administrators. In the early 1990s, persons from these disciplines got together to design a hospital unit that would be elder-friendly in order to prevent functional decline in frail older adults beyond what would be expected by their acute illness or injury (Landefeld, Palmer, Kresevic, Fortinsky, & Kowal, 1995; Palmer, Landefeld, Kresevic, & Kowal, 1994).

The professionals described above observed that elders often demonstrated severe functional decline caused by stressors associated with hospitalization. Some of those stressors were tethers such as intravenous (IV) lines, foley catheters, and nasogastric (NG) tubes; prolonged bedrest; dependence on hospital staff for toileting, eating, taking fluids, and ambulation; new medications and/or anesthesia; confusing stimuli in the environment; poor lighting; low toilet seats; lack of sensory aides; isolation; and fragmented care. Because many elders were in frail health prior to their acute illness or injury, these added hospital stressors plus the reason for their hospitalization put them "over the edge" of their functional abilities.

Very soon, these frail elders became incapacitated in the hospital setting and were no longer able to return to their homes. Therefore, the purpose for establishing the first ACE unit, and for measuring outcomes compared to usual care, was twofold: (a) to demonstrate that functional decline could be prevented, and (b) to demonstrate cost effectiveness of the ACE protocols.

Interdisciplinary Conferences

The ACE model of care is interdisciplinary and low-tech. Persons who were randomized into the ACE group had their care reviewed daily in team conferences led by a clinical nurse specialist (CNS) with expertise in gerontology. Other attendees were the medical director for ACE, the patient's primary nurse, a pharmacologist and physical therapist, and others if needed, such as a psychiatrist, family member(s), or attending physician. The interdisciplinary team identified risk factors or developing problems for each ACE patient, decided on treatments or interventions to reduce those risk factors or problems, and wrote suggestions for physicians' orders on a yellow sheet that was placed in the patient's chart in the section marked progress notes. Attending physicians were asked to initial the suggestions and indicate "agree" or "disagree" (with a reason for not implementing the suggestion in the progress notes) (Panno, Kolcaba, & Holder, 2000).

Environment

An important part of any ACE unit were environmental adaptations that enabled the units to be more elder-friendly. Innovations included handrails along all hallways, door handles that arthritic hands could push open, nonglare but high intensity lighting, large calendars and clocks in every room, soothing and noninstitutional color on walls and floors, family lounge and dining areas where patients could congregate, and carpet squares on all floors to provide nonslip surfaces. Such modifications made it easier for older patients to adapt to the hospital stay.

Medical Director and Clinical Nurse Specialist

In the early stages of the pilot study, the medical director for ACE was essential as a liaison between the interdisciplinary team and attending physicians. He had received specialized education in geriatric medicine, preparing him for multiple roles such as educator, researcher, and counselor. The medical director spent much time discussing the suggestions of the interdisciplinary team with the patients' private doctors and, if a doctor was hesitant about implementing a suggestion, discussed the full range of comments that emanated from team conferences. Soon, the attending physicians found that their patients were doing better when the suggestions of the ACE team were implemented (Panno, Kolcaba, & Holder, 2000) and asked that their elderly patients be placed on ACE units in the future.

The clinical nurse specialist (CNS) convened the interdisciplinary conferences every day, calling together the primary nurses who cared for ACE patients, and making arrangements for special guests, such as family members, to attend. She carefully reviewed the charts of ACE patients prior to the meetings, noting progress regarding problems or risk factors that had been identified. She served as a support and resource person to nurses and other personnel involved with the ACE patients, and kept track of recommendations and concerns of students and family members. These would be discussed in the next team conference.

Nurse Initiated Guidelines

Another departure from usual care were guidelines for nurse initiated protocols that could be implemented by nurses without physicians' orders. Thus, nurses on the ACE unit, who had 8 hours of in-house continuing education, had a more autonomous practice with increased accountability. Preventive and restorative nursing guidelines focused on activities of daily living (ADLs), mobility, toileting, nutrition and hydration, skin care, patient safety, and treatment of acute confusion or depression. Guidelines included goals and suggested nursing interventions that could be individualized and implemented without physicians' orders such as bedside commodes, toileting schedules, screening for depression and dementia, removal of mechanical restraints, insertion of heparin locks, or skin care interventions. Such interventions were evaluated during interdisciplinary conferences (Panno, Kolcaba, & Holder, 2000; Palmer, Landefeld, Kresevic, & Kowal, 1994).

Home Discharge Planning

The interdisciplinary team initiated discharge assessments and plans upon admission. Plans for special equipment, home adaptations, home nursing or aides, therapies, medication management, meals, and doctors' appointments were high priorities. Family members were consulted and supported in planning for discharge. When patients came into the hospital *from* home, the goal was to return them to home (Panno, Kolcaba, & Holder, 2000).

Follow-up Contacts

After discharge, the CNS phoned the ACE patients using an interdisciplinary communication sheet to follow up on functional or psychosocial problems/risk factors identified during the hospital stay. The communication sheets were also used by home nurses to carry out the plan of care in the home setting. Calls from the CNS were made to physicians when necessary to modify medications at home or order additional supports. This follow-up process was instrumental in preventing immediate and costly readmissions.

Comfort Care

A holistic perspective was inherent in the ACE model. Students utilized Comfort Theory to assess patients' physical, emotional, spiritual, social, cultural and environmental needs within the context of home and family. The CNS brought these components together during interdisciplinary conferences in order to plan for and implement holistic hospital care and discharge planning. Because patients' comfort was enhanced through nursing care, their progress in rehabilitation was enhanced (Panno, Kolcaba, & Holder, 2000). A model of Comfort Care was not built into the project's design because the development phase occurred prior to my thinking about outcomes research. The CNS told us, though, that being educated about holistic assessment is an essential ingredient for the team members.

Research

In order to demonstrate that ACE principles and holistic care worked, outcomes research was conducted. ACE began in Cleveland, Ohio and the pilot study there showed that patients who were randomized into the ACE protocols were more functional at discharge than patients discharged from a traditional unit (Landefeld et al., 1995). Because of these promising results, the study was repeated in a larger population in Cleveland and Akron, Ohio. The latter site was where I was doing my clinical supervision of junior-level nursing students and we were privileged to be a part of their demonstration project.

Over the first 9 months of the study, 161 patients 70 years of age or older were assigned to ACE protocols and 165 patients to usual care. All patients were similar in sociodemographic characteristics, functional status, and coexisting illnesses (Panno, Kolcaba, & Holder, 2000). Some of the findings were these: (a) ACE patients had 0.8 days shorter length of stay and cost $1,490.00 less than patients discharged from other units, a savings of $1.3 million in 9 months; (b) ACE patients received significantly more care plans for mobility, continence, and falls prevention; (c) restraints were less often applied with no increase in falls; (d) discharge planning was initiated earlier; (e) physicians, nurses, families, and patients were more satisfied with care on the ACE unit; and (f) physicians more often rated the ACE unit as excellent in meeting the needs of older patients, planning for discharge, providing the reporting physicians with useful information, and implementing treatment plans (Panno, Kolcaba, & Holder, 2000).

While the above outcomes were impressive, nursing-sensitive outcomes were not measured. Such outcomes as enhanced comfort and its relationship to faster healing, increased progress in physical therapy, and patients' feelings of confidence, determination, and motivation would be more discipline specific for nursing (Figure 9.1). Also, the *comfort of nurses* was essential to the success of the project. This unit provided support for their efforts, education about new strategies for care, and requested feedback about what did and did not work to improve patient outcomes. Such comfort measures for nurses are important to measure because they are related to cost savings achieved through higher nurse retention and attendance.

3. Parish Nursing

Parish nursing is an evolving and rapidly growing specialty in nursing with standards of practice issued in 1998 by the American Nurses Association and the Health Ministries Association, Inc. The Scope and Standards of Parish Nursing addresses the

> independent practice of professional nursing, as defined by the nursing practice act in each state, in health promotion within the context of the client's values, beliefs, and faith practices. Spiritual care is a major component of health promotion activities. The client focus is the faith community, including its families and individual members and the community it serves. (American Nurses Association and the Health Ministries Association, Inc., 1998, p. 2)

Parish nursing began as a grassroots, ecumenical movement in the United States in which nurses focus their attention on the spiritual and physical health of parishioners. In a variety of ways, parish nurses promote health education and restoration, the mind-body-spirit connection, and the prevention of disease and injury. They assist parishioners with negotiating the maze of health care when symptoms arise, receiving essential social supports and referrals, and integrating spirituality into health issues. Parish nurses organize health fairs and screenings and teach classes on such topics as stress reduction, weight control, living wills, suicide prevention, grief, and loss. They publish health information in church newsletters. Some act as counselors, visiting congregation members in their homes, nursing homes, or in hospitals. Often, they teach individuals the proper use of medications, explain medical terminology, go to doctors' appointments with individuals, or make referrals to resources in the community.

Nursing care is delivered within the structures of organized places of worship. Some nurses have scheduled office hours within their houses of worship, where they provide a place for patients to talk about the deeper issues in life that have an impact on their health. Having an office with posted hours helps establish a visible presence for the congregation.

Parish nurses take professional practice into faith communities as health educators, health counselors, teachers of volunteers, and liaisons to other health agencies. They can work within their own congregations or with other congregations. Parish nurses do not provide "hands-on" care as do home care nurses, but when congregation members are ineligible for home care services or cannot get out for screenings or doctors' appointments, parish nurses or volunteers pick up the slack by visiting those members who can't get out. As the gap widens between what services are covered by insurance such as Medicare and those services actually needed in the community, partnering with faith communities provides a vital link to the health care delivery system and enhances the health status of participating congregations. The parish nurse is in a position to positively influence congregations to be good stewards of their bodies and to teach them to nurture self-worth and their inherent value (Westberg, 1990).

History

Parish nursing traces its roots to the early deaconesses called to Christian service in the early 1800s. Parish nursing of today evolved from the work of Dr. Granger Westberg, a hospital chaplain and professor. Westberg believed that to make the behavioral changes needed for health promotion and disease prevention, persons needed to be motivated, this motivation coming from a person's outlook on life. He believed that persons' philosophy of life along with their belief system and faith could provide needed motivation for change. Further, he believed that whole-person care in centers where a doctor, nurse, and pastor worked as a team would make a significant difference in prevention of illness and disease (Westberg, 1990).

With support of the W. K. Kellogg Foundation, Westberg established 12 family doctor offices in church buildings. These centers became teaching centers for medical students, nursing students, and pastors from across the United States and Canada. After the project was completed, Westberg continued the parish nurse model, combining the skills of the pastor and the registered nurse in health promotion and disease prevention. In his book, Westberg states,

> Nurses are national treasures, reservoirs of compassion and strength, and pearls of great price that have been hidden from view for far too long. For more than 40 years nurses have pleaded with the medical profession that it become more oriented toward preventive medicine, that it concentrate on teaching people how to stay well. Now is their chance to reach thousands of people in the informal setting of an institution that is ready to rethink its role in motivating people toward healthy living. (Westberg, 1990, p. 20)

Four common models for delivery of parish nurse care are:

1. Nurse is employed by a health care system/institution that provides liability insurance and owns its own records for clients seen.
2. Nurse is employed by the congregation who pays for liability insurance and owns the records for clients seen.
3. Nurse is not compensated (volunteers) and obtains his or her own liability insurance. Either the nurse or the congregation owns the records for clients seen.
4. Nurse has a contractual arrangement between a health care system (HCS) and congregation, where the HCS provides liability insurance, consulting, and the congregation assists with payment for the nurse and services.

The International Parish Nurse Resource Center (IPNRC; 1999) in St. Louis, Missouri, provides support and training for parish nurses. The course curriculum is owned by the Resource Center and is taught throughout the country. It is endorsed by both the National League for Nursing and the American Nurses Association. It can be taught for 3 hours of college credit or 31 continuing education units. The Resource Center also provides an annual and inspiring 3-day conference for continuing education for parish nurses and it has a Website.

Comfort Care in Parish Nursing

The framework of comfort care for Parish Nursing (Figure 9.4) guides my small group of parish nurses in several ways. First, it directs us to assess holistic needs of our members and friends in four contexts of comfort (physical, psychospiritual, sociocultural, and environmental). While formal needs assessments are available, nurses can supplement those findings with observations made informally. For example, I am a member of our Elderlife board and became aware that drivers using church vans to transport seniors to social events were not requiring the use of seat belts. Our of parish nurses signed a letter of support for repair or replacement of existing seat belts and to stipulate that seat belts should be installed for future purchases of vans. We also recommended installation of signs in each van asking users to "buckle up." This intervention was intended to improve the environmental and social comfort (i.e., safety) of elders using the vans.

Secondly, the Comfort Care framework reminds us to identify intervening variables of congregations that will impact on chosen interventions. Such intervening variables might be socioeconomic status of the

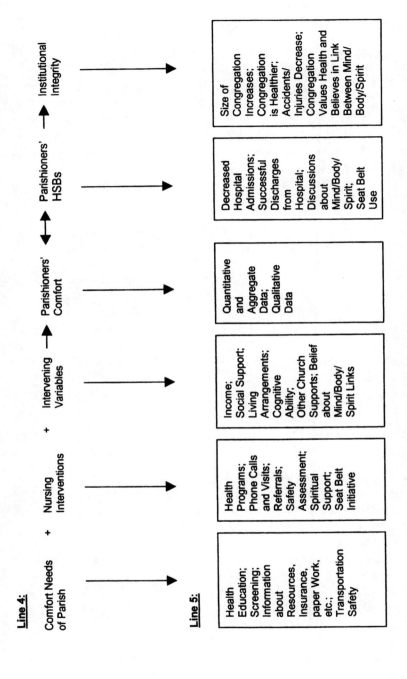

Line 4:

Comfort Needs of Parish + Nursing Interventions + Intervening Variables → Parishioners' Comfort ↔ Parishioners' HSBs → Institutional Integrity

Line 5:

| Health Education; Screening; Information about Resources, Insurance, paper Work, etc.; Transportation Safety | Health Programs; Phone Calls and Visits; Referrals; Safety Assessment; Spiritual Support; Seat Belt Initiative | Income; Social Support; Living Arrangements; Cognitive Ability; Other Church Supports; Belief about Mind/Body/ Spirit Links | Quantitative and Aggregate Data; Qualitative Data | Decreased Hospital Admissions; Successful Discharges from Hospital; Discussions about Mind/Body/ Spirit; Seat Belt Use | Size of Congregation Increases; Congregation is Healthier; Accidents/ Injuries Decrease; Congregation Values Health and Believes in Link Between Mind/ Body/Spirit |

FIGURE 9.4 Theoretical framework for parish nursing.

congregation, demographics of members, availability of transportation and other community supports, extent of volunteer programs, etc. Third, HSBs of the congregation are indicators of short-term outcomes, such as engaging in health promoting activities, healing well after surgery, or peaceful deaths of members when that is the most realistic outcome. Fourth, institutional outcomes can be measured with group data such as incidence of hospitalizations, emergency department visits, serious injuries, etc.

Documentation

Because many parish nurses have collaborative practices with hospitals, charting has become an important issue. Hospitals must comply with Joint Commission American Hospital Organization (JCAHO) regulations about charting. In addition, parish nurses must document patient outcomes so that their practice in the community is validated.

Currently, the IPNRC advocates the use of the NIC and NOC classification systems for use in documenting interventions and outcomes of all parish nurses. In their publications, forms and instructions are included for charting using NIC and NOC, and for several nursing diagnoses related to spiritual care. Comfort, already listed in NOC, is an important outcome of parish nursing practice, especially when nurses use Comfort Care for their practice framework.

4. Community Comfort Care

Community health-public health (CH-PH) nursing synthesizes community nursing principles with a population-based approach. Settings in which CH-PH nurses practice include state health departments, visiting nurse services, community or neighborhood health centers, and day care centers among others. CH-PH nursing addresses issues such as teen pregnancy, student health, substance abuse and homelessness (Kovner, Harrington, & Mezey, 2001). Most baccalaureate nursing programs and RN degree programs provide specific education in CH-PH nursing. This educational focus can also be found in graduate nursing programs as well as in schools of public health.

The government document, *Healthy People 2010* (U.S. Department of Health and Human Services, 2000, p. 2), usually guides curriculum development, students' papers and presentations, and their clinical experiences. According to this far-reaching document, two overarching goals for health in the United States by the year 2010 are to (a) increase quality and years of healthy life, and (b) eliminate health disparities (p. 2).

Also within *Healthy People 2010* are listed 28 focus areas for health education and intervention (Table 9.1). Students, educators, and researchers can pick from among these focus areas, topics for in-depth consideration and development of class projects and/or proposals.

The CH-PH course that I helped teach was an RN-BSN completion course in which students spent considerable time doing community assessments. As they did this project, they were asked to identify comfort needs related to either of the above two goals and at least one of the 28 focus areas. We adapted Comfort Theory for CH-PH nursing, utilizing community nursing concepts as much as possible. The care plan that students used for their assignment is depicted in Figure 9.5. Care plans were then completed by the students that reflected for nursing care of groups within the community.

Line 4 in Figure 9.6 is analogous to all of the line 4s in other figures presented. It is the mid-range theory level. Line 5 in Figure 9.6 shows

TABLE 9.1 Healthy People 2010 Focus Areas

1. Access to Quality Health Services	15. Injury and Violence Prevention
2. Arthritis, Osteoporosis, and Chronic Back Conditions	16. Maternal, Infant, and Child Health
3. Cancer	17. Medical Product Safety
4. Chronic Kidney Disease	18. Mental Health and Mental Disorders
5. Diabetes	
6. Disability and Secondary Conditions	19. Nutrition and Overweight
	20. Occupational Safety and Health
7. Educational and Community-Based Programs	21. Oral Health
	22. Physical Activity and Fitness
8. Environmental Health	23. Public Health Infrastructure
9. Family Planning	24. Respiratory Diseases
10. Food Safety	25. Sexually Transmitted Diseases
11. Health Communication	26. Substance Abuse
12. Heart Disease and Stroke	27. Tobacco Use
13. HIV	28. Vision and Hearing
14. Immunization and Infectious Diseases	

Reprinted from *Healthy People 2010: Understanding and Improving Health* (2nd ed.). Washington, DC: U.S. Department of Health and Human Services.

Nurse/Student Name _____

Population _____

Assessment (Health/Comfort Needs)	Policy Development (Intervention)	Intervening Variables	Identified Comfort Needs Met (Immediate Outcome)	Assurance HSB/Subsequent Outcomes	Long-Term Community Effect
Physical					
Psychospiritual					
Sociocultural					
Environmental					

FIGURE 9.5 Care plan for community Comfort Care.

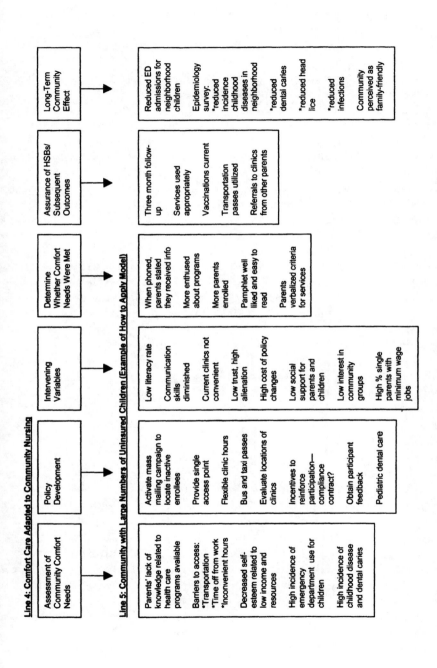

FIGURE 9.6 Theoretical framework for Comfort Care in the community.

Line 4: Comfort Care Adapted to Community Nursing

Assessment of Community Comfort Needs	Policy Development	Intervening Variables	Determine Whether Comfort Needs Were Met	Assurance of HSBs/ Subsequent Outcomes	Long-Term Community Effect

Line 5: Community with Large Numbers of Uninsured Children (Example of How to Apply Model)

Assessment of Community Comfort Needs	Policy Development	Intervening Variables	Determine Whether Comfort Needs Were Met	Assurance of HSBs/ Subsequent Outcomes	Long-Term Community Effect
Parents' lack of knowledge related to health care programs available	Activate mass mailing campaign to locate inactive enrollees	Low literacy rate	When phoned, parents stated they received info	Three month follow-up	Reduced ED admissions for neighborhood children
Barriers to access: *Transportation *Time off from work *Inconvenient hours	Provide single access point Flexible clinic hours	Communication skills diminished Current clinics not convenient	More enthused about programs More parents enrolled	Services used appropriately Vaccinations current	Epidemiology survey: *reduced incidence childhood diseases in neighborhood
Decreased self-esteem related to low income and resources	Bus and taxi passes Evaluate locations of clinics	Low trust, high alienation High cost of policy changes	Pamphlet well liked and easy to read	Transportation passes utilized Referrals to clinics from other parents	*reduced dental caries
High incidence of emergency department use for children	Incentives to reinforce participation—compliance contract?	Low social support for parents and children Low interest in community groups	Parents verbalized criteria for services		*reduced head lice *reduced infections
High incidence of childhood disease and dental caries	Obtain participant feedback Pediatric dental care	High % single parents with minimum wage jobs			Community perceived as family-friendly

179

how the concepts in Line 4 were operationalized by five students working together on their community assessment. The community that they assessed was a small, rural community in Ohio. All of the students were asked to pick a community different from where they lived. The target population of the example was medically uninsured children. I publish this work with the students' permission.

Adapting from the expanded framework for the Theory of Comfort, comfort needs were conceptualized as those factors in the community that detracted from the citizens' health, safety, or empowerment. Students were asked to think about physical, psychospiritual, sociocultural, and environmental comfort needs evident in their communities of study. Eventually they narrowed down the total picture of community comfort needs to one smaller area for attention, and focused their care plans on a specific health issue explicated in *Healthy People 2010* (U.S. Department of Health and Human Services, 2000). In this case, the focus was on improving children's access to health care.

Students listed their findings from the assessment under the heading of "Assessment of Community Comfort Needs." The term interventions was restated as "policy development" and students listed actions that CH-PH nurses could take to help pediatric clinics achieve better utilization by their target population. Intervening variables were those factors over which nurses or the clinics had little control, but which could affect the direction and success of their care plan. Nurses determined whether comfort needs were met in the target population by gathering objective, subjective, and supporting data. Under health seeking behaviors, nurses listed goals that were realistic for their population. The concept of Institutional Integrity (InI) was changed to "Long-Term Community Effect" to accommodate the community setting. Thus, desired effects of the new policies that the students developed were listed under this last column.

The faculty teaching this course were happy with the results of the community care plans that the students produced. In addition, we asked the students to evaluate the usefulness of Comfort Theory for doing community assessments. They responded positively with remarks such as: "Thinking about factors that make a community a comfortable one to live in was really challenging;" "Comfort Theory helped me to think about the community holistically. I thought about physical, psychospiritual, social, cultural, and environmental comfort with safety being a part of social and environmental comfort;" and "This was a different way to think about the living conditions of certain communities. Everyone wants to be comfortable where they live."

It is indeed interesting to think about holistic comfort needs that are present because of the structure of communities. *Physical* comfort needs pertain to the quality of air, water, streets, and noise level. *Psycho-spiritual* comfort needs pertain to the extent of participation/marginalization of community members and the presence of houses of worship congruent with the population. *Sociocultural* comfort needs relate to the extent of social support available, educational and income levels of residents, openness to diversity, and tolerance for diverse cultural traditions. *Environmental* comfort needs pertain to safety issues, such as presence of violence, safe railroad crossings, sidewalks, playgrounds, lighting, transportation, support for older adults in their homes, access to health care, presence and approachability of police and firefighters, appearance of homes and buildings, logical and pleasing zoning, green spaces, etc. The total picture regarding these factors and others are strong indicators of the health and quality of life of citizens in any given community, whether they are young, old, or in between. From our Nightingale heritage to *Healthy People 2010*, nurses have a mandate to assume a leadership role for improving the environment within our communities.

COMFORT OF NURSES

Prior to writing this book, I had done only a little thinking about the comfort of nurses—in fact, I focused deliberately on patient comfort because I believe that the documentation and measurement of positive patient outcomes is the essence of the science of nursing care. When I first encountered the second quote for this chapter, however, it caused me to pause. That pause was reinforced by the current projections of shortages in hospital nurses. Nurses *do* perform difficult and stressful jobs in the hospitals, with little or no reward or recognition. I agree with the American Nurses Association that there isn't a real nursing shortage (yet), it's just that nurses have left their hospital positions in droves, sick and tired of the poor working conditions. As some would say, nurses vote with their feet.

I now work under the assumption that realities associated with hospital environments are the essence of the science of nursing administration. I also believe that the holistic comfort of nurses is an important factor in retention, absenteeism, morale, and recruitment. To assist my thinking about this reality and how nurse administrators might ap-

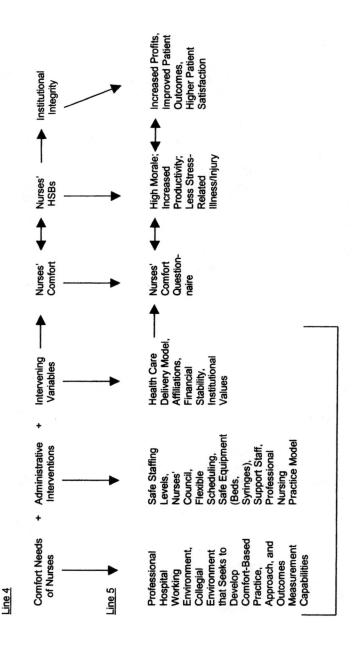

FIGURE 9.7 Theoretical framework for a study of nurses' comfort.

Line 4

Comfort Needs + Administrative + Intervening ⟶ Nurses' ⟷ Nurses' ⟶ Institutional
of Nurses   Interventions   Variables   Comfort   HSBs   Integrity

Line 5

| Professional Hospital Working Environment, Collegial Environment that Seeks to Develop Comfort-Based Practice, Approach, and Outcomes Measurement Capabilities | Safe Staffing Levels, Nurses' Council, Flexible Scheduling, Safe Equipment (Beds, Syringes), Support Staff, Professional Nursing Practice Model | Health Care Delivery Model, Affiliations, Financial Stability, Institutional Values | Nurses' Comfort Question-naire | High Morale; Increased Productivity; Less Stress-Related Illness/Injury | Increased Profits, Improved Patient Outcomes, Higher Patient Satisfaction |

Line 6 This is the operational level. Line 5 consists of suggestions, not all of which can be implemented at one time. What interventions and nurse outcomes is YOUR institution or nurse administrator interested in? What indicators of InI are relevant and possible to measure? The possibilities are endless. Good luck!

proach it, I drew yet another comfort diagram (I guess I think better with diagrams). In Figure 9.7, specific comfort needs such as safe equipment, improved wages and benefits, and flexible family-friendly scheduling are subsumed under "professional working environment." Nurses want input on decisions affecting staffing, assignments, and the model of care delivery. They want autonomy to practice to their fullest and they want respect for their contributions. Lack of attention to these important workplace issues is, I believe, the root of the nursing shortage. As well, addressing the comfort needs of nurses and other members of the health care team is essential for improving patient care and for maintaining the integrity of the institution. Comfort Care offers a positive, holistic, logical model for potential magnet organizations (American Nurses Association, 2001). Much work is left to be done in getting the word out, as we all know.

MUSINGS ON COMFORT QUOTE (CHAPTER 9)

> First and foremost, human beings—worldwide—want to be comforted and kept safe by nursing care.
> —M. Mallison, Editor, *American Journal of Nursing*, 1990, p. 15

I chose this quotes because it illustrates an important goal that I have in writing this book. First, I want to highlight the important mission that nurses have been given by their public—to comfort their patients in times of health-related stress. Patients intuitively know that comfort is a strengthening tool that needs to be used for coping and healing. They know that there are comfort needs that cannot be met by family members because of the highly technical and changing exigencies in the health care arena. Therefore, patients rely on nurses to be their advocates, their source of understandable information, and their resource for further services as needed. Of all the health care personnel available, patients trust nurses most (Malone, 1999)—we, as a discipline, must give patients what they want, need, and expect in order to maintain that high level of trust.

> We labour soon, we labour late to feed the titled knave, man;
> And ah, the comfort we're to get, is that beyond the grave, man.
> —Robert Burns, Scottish poet (1838), *The Tree of Liberty*

This quote speaks to the comfort of nurses, another important goal for this book. I certainly hope that nurses' comfort becomes valued in our lifetime—the comfort to practice holistically, the comfort of a professional hospital environment in which to work, the comfort of having predictable schedules that give reverence to family and professional life, the comfort of being supported by administrators in terms of benefits, salaries, pensions, and continuing education. These comforts are basic, modest, and not uncommon compared with other professions, but have eluded nurses for many reasons. May this be *our* time for being strengthened through comfort—and may we receive professional comfort before the grave!

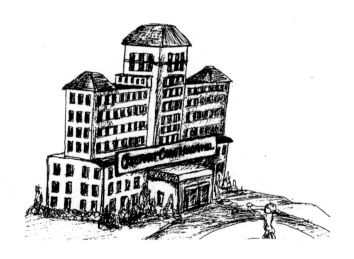

CHAPTER 10

Visions of Comfort
for the Future

On Tuesday, September 11, 2001, the future of the United States and perhaps the world was drastically altered. We were plunged into the unknown, from which we will create a new future. My visions of comfort were impacted greatly by this cataclysmic event, and I share some comfort quotes about this event because they hint at possible new directions for comfort care.

> Across the nation Friday [September 14, 2001], people gathered to comfort each other during a national day of prayer. . . . Participants joined hands for a moment of silence.
> —Brazaitis, T., "The survivors need help too." *Cleveland Plain Dealer*, Sunday, September 16, 2001, p. H-3

> We said I love you a thousand times over and over again, and it just brought so much peace to us," says Lyz [wife of Jeremy Glick, hero on Flight 93 out of Newark, which crashed in Pennsylvania on September 11, 2001]. "I felt the feeling from it. He told me, "I love Emmy"—who is our daughter—"and to take care of her." Then he said, "Whatever decisions you make in your life, I need you to be happy, and I will respect any decisions that you make."

That's what he said and that gives me the most comfort.
He sounded strong. He didn't sound panicked, very clear-
headed. I told him to put a picture of me and Emmy in
his head to be strong. . . . And then he said, "I need some
advice . . . we're talking about attacking these men, what
should I do?" And then I finally just decided at that instant
that "Honey, you need to do it."
—Elyzabeth Glick (wife of Jeremy Glick) interviewed by
Jane Pauley on Dateline, NBC, September 18, 2001

"I think about the families, the children," the President
told reporters gathered in the Oval Office, looking away
for a moment to compose himself. "I wish I could comfort
every single family whose lives have been affected."
—George W. Bush, as reported by Bob Kemper,
Chicago Tribune, September 14, 2001, pp. 1–3

Dzemila Spahovic is a case manager with the refugee mental
health program reporting about her nightmares Tuesday
night, after the attack on America. "When I came here, I
hoped we would stay safe for all time," she said as she
counsels Bosnians who are confused, unable to sleep, and
afraid of sudden noises. Spahovic said it can be difficult to
offer comfort while haunted by her own fears. "But," she
said, smiling. "Somebody has to do it."
—Dzemila Spahovic, as reported by J. Lieblich and
S. Franklin, *Chicago Tribune*, September 14, 2001, pp. 1–11

Our national tragedy occurred just 5 days ago, as I was preparing mentally to begin this chapter. Needless to say, that event changed this last
chapter in ways that I couldn't have predicted. That Tuesday began
like any other U.S. workday, and along the East coast (where New York
City and Washington, D.C. are located), the skies were brilliantly blue
and the temperature delightful. At 8:45 AM, however, as workers were
getting into their offices, a passenger jet slammed into the north tower
of the World Trade Center. Fifteen minutes later, a second jet plowed
into the south tower and, shortly after that, a third jet into the Pentagon
in Washington, D.C.

At about the same time as the Pentagon crash, a fourth hijacked
plane entered the airspace over my home city of Cleveland, Ohio, and
then abruptly turned around to take aim at the nation's capitol in

Washington, D.C. That fourth set of hijackers was overtaken by five brave passengers on the plane and it crashed in a Pennsylvania field. Two hundred passengers and crew members were lost in the four planes and over 2,100 fire fighters, police, and civilians were lost on the ground. It was a horrific event in scope and violation.

In the news articles and commentaries spoken and written since, we learned of heroics and heartbreaks of staggering dimensions. We also learned afresh how much we loved our country and each other. As I gradually turned from television to contemplation, I became aware again of comfort as a prominent need and a prominent behavior of caring people. Why is that? And how is it that we all intuit it's meaning, no matter how it is used? The richness and versatility of this concept continue to amaze me, and I am proud that nursing embraced comfort as a mission more than 100 years ago. The quotes above tell us not to forget about the importance of comfort and comforting in this crazy world of ours. Truly, comfort is needed now more than ever.

In this chapter, I will explore with you the importance of comfort as a universal communicator and fortifier. I will attempt to create a new vision for how we, as health care providers, can renew our mission of providing comfort to our patients, so that they can engage more fully in health seeking behaviors (HSBs). Comfort will be discussed at five levels: the patient/family level; the hospital/agency level; the local community level; the national level; and the global level. I have thought about the first three levels for some years now. But the Attack on America, so fresh in my mind, has compelled me to try to address the ideas of national and global comfort. Thus, in the next pages, I will attempt to provide some insight into what those ideals of national comfort and global comfort might mean. I hope you will permit me to dream and create a "mythic vision" (Berry, 1988) for Comfort Care in the future. As Dzemila Spahovic said above about providing comfort in the midst of duress and change, "Somebody has to do it."

COMFORT AT THE PATIENT/FAMILY LEVEL

In the future, I am hopeful that comfort of individuals and families in any health care setting will be valued highly, whether caregivers are physicians, social workers, pharmacists, physical therapists, or nurses. Nurses can lead the way in bringing patient/family comfort back into the consciousnesses of health care providers so that the specter of being hospitalized for illness or injury looms less dangerous and frightening. Comfort Care, as a model for health care delivery, can be promoted as one that has universal appeal, ease of use, intuitive familiarity, and subsequent benefits for recipients as well as institutions.

Nurses must continue to promote health and safety through vaccinations, helmet and seat belt usage, and informed lifestyle choices so that our own neighbors and family members stay healthier longer. We will be more credible if we role model these health practices and values and the way we treat each other. We can "look out" for each other in our communities, while being vigilant and thoughtful about what is happening in the outer world.

We *must* become proactive. We have in this country a shameful percentage of adults and children who have no help with their health care costs or worse, no homes at all. The problem of children and adults who are uninsured or homeless is a nursing problem that is so mired in politics and economics that we feel almost hopeless to facilitate change. We must believe strongly that everyone has a right to basic health services and basic comforts such as food, clothing, education, social kindness, and shelter. We must also advocate for those who are disenfranchised by becoming political ourselves and trying to be part of the process of equitable change.

While serving those who are homeless and/or uninsured, we also need to express our outrage that such inequities exist. We can be advocates by writing letters to editors, running for political office, voting and encouraging the disenfranchised to vote, joining professional organizations, and speaking to our legislators. As the Universal Declaration of Human Rights, written by the United Nations, states: "People have duties towards the place where they live and towards other people who live there with them" (United Nations, 2000). Many nurses have left the hospital setting, but we cannot abandon our duties as nurses to advocate for fair treatment, health, and comfort of our fellow life-travelers in our communities, cities, and countries. We comfort each other by holding hands and recognizing that we are all in this fight together. Nurses just might be the best persons to articulate what the fight in health care is about—we are trusted, we are plentiful, and we care. Although our voices are small and disparate presently, through our own comfort with each other and our professional roles, we will be strengthened to shout out together what needs to be done!

COMFORT AT THE HOSPITAL/INSTITUTIONAL LEVEL

Ten years ago, economists specializing in health care predicted that hospitals would undergo radical reductions in occupancy and many would close. A rise in home care would be the logical result, with the reasoning being that most people preferred to be cared for in their homes, given enough support. Presently, in 2002, some community hospitals are closed, but most were swallowed up by large conglomerates.

These conglomerate hospital groups are still competing for business in a variety of costly ways, such as marketing, building new structures, and buying expensive equipment. In the meantime, reimbursement for home care has been slashed by Congress. Presently, health care costs are higher than ever, access to health care is uneven, and one serious illness or injury can leave a patient or family destitute. Where, oh where, is the altruism in this business?

Nurses are currently advocating for changes in staffing and working conditions in hospitals, under the mantra of patient safety. Safety to me, while important, seems to entail a minimum level of care—it seems to say, "If you are a patient at this hospital, you will not get hurt." Such a standard is hardly a goal for best care. Best care means that patients and families are kept comfortable so they feel strengthened to heal and engage in HSBs. Healing, in turn, refers to what the patient needs to do at any given time, including feeling empowered to die peacefully or let a loved one go. The large percentage of health care dollars that are spent on patients who are dying would be reduced to a more reasonable figure if hospital care focused on comfort and healing. A vision that I hold is that hospitals will gradually become places where decisions are guided by this kind of thinking.

Another reason for adopting patient comfort as a goal for nursing care is that it is subjective and other directed. That is, we all know when we are comfortable. Patients also know when they are comfortable, or at least more comfortable than they were before nursing interventions. Neither we nor our patients can know much about our own safety—the wave of terrorism across our country demonstrates that we, and our patients, can only hope for safety. Because comfort is subjective, it is measurable and it is patient focused.

One of my mythic visions for the future of hospital care is that administrators will begin to advocate for the comfort of their patients. Think about how appealing the following slogan might be as an advertising tool: "We are a Comfort Care hospital." Such a slogan could be used for recruitment of nurses as well as patients and their insurers! Hospitals that make explicit their interest in providing comfort to patients, through taking measures that make nurses comfortable, will have no shortage of patients or nurses. Insurers want to be affiliated with hospitals that make their insurees feel better. In addition, men and women want to be in helping professions where their creativity and caring are valued and respected—by bosses and patients.

For the hospital of tomorrow, Comfort Care is a framework for practicing holistically, as most of us learned to do in school (Kolcaba, 2000). This is a nursing ideal, but to accomplish it requires time and energy, focus, and positive reinforcement. The full job description of nursing has to include attention to whole patients with a statement such as, "The nurse will address the holistic needs of patients and their families, including physical, psychospiritual, sociocultural, and environmental needs."

In a Comfort Care hospital, the goal of holistic interdisciplinary care (and it is important to have a measurable goal) is to enhance comfort for patients assigned to our care. To accomplish this, nurses need continuity in assignments so that, through comfort, we can bring the strengths of our patients and families to bear on their own health issues. We need a formal structure for bringing the interdisciplinary team together to discuss how best to prevent functional decline and optimize discharge planning. We need time to get to know our patients, and to assess their holistic comfort needs. We need an environment that supports us as human beings who need to eat, rest, and return to our families as scheduled. We need benefits, roles, and respect congruent with other highly educated professionals. Changes such as these are congruent with the ideals of magnet hospitals described in chapter 9 (American Nurses Association, 2001).

Perhaps nurses in Comfort Care hospitals would manage their own units through bottom-up management, in which workers vote on everything including whether a new co-worker gets permanently hired and how the group schedules lunch breaks (Simon, 1999). Professionals and nonprofessionals on each unit test models and vote on best methods for scheduling, budgeting, assigning patient care, team-leading, rewarding workers, and so forth. Models that "fit" and are cost effective, morale improving, retention producing, and comfort enhancing (for patients and nurses) are maintained and become role models for other units (Kolcaba, 2000).

Comfort Care hospitals would measure productivity in terms of the patients' progress in the hospital and at home. These hospitals would subscribe to the belief that the nursing-sensitive outcome of comfort contributes to multidisciplinary outcomes such as successful discharge and patient satisfaction (as seen in Figure 9.2). Comfort Care hospitals would then facilitate and measure patient comfort as well as global measures. Relationships between patient comfort and subsequent multidisciplinary measures would be assessed. This hospital would then have evidence for the benefits of strong nursing models and policies that in turn encourage retention and productivity. Patients would heal faster, and hospitals' "bottom line" would benefit. My vision is a "win-win" proposition. As well, designation as a magnet organization provides further incentive in the form of grant programs for those so designated.

COMFORT AT THE COMMUNITY LEVEL

My mythic vision for Comfort Care in the community is even more idealistic! It includes a community that has mechanisms for supporting patients and their families at home after their early discharges from cost-saving hospitals. Such supports might be in the form of parish nurses, care managers, social workers, nursing assistants, and physicians who provide services in patients' homes. Interventions for comfort would actually be reimbursable! The interdisciplinary teams would be housed centrally within the communities that they serve. Within these community offices, models of care delivery again would be developed from the bottom up, with holistic and affordable care the common goal. Perhaps consumers could have some choices among providers, based on personality, fees, and success rates. (This assumes that larger communities, especially, will have more than one holistic health team.)

I read that in Japan, healthy neighbors and acquaintances receive credits for helping sick or frail neighbors in their homes with transportation, cooking, shopping, dressing, bathing, banking, recreation, home upkeep, and companionship. At a central community office, these credits (we could call them Comfort Credits) are tallied, recorded, and filed every week or so. When that Comfort Worker, in turn, becomes sick or frail (s)he cashes in the credits that were earned in the past and a new Comfort Worker starts earning Comfort Credits. There is some appeal to this mutual aid method, although it seems a bit calculated to me. But better to have a system of banking Comfort Credits for later payback than to ignore the needs of frail and ill neighbors within our own communities.

Another health issue that needs to be looked at in the community is to identify and work toward factors that make a community comfortable. Such factors might be sidewalks, safe intersections and crossings for pedestrians, public transportation, proximity of essential services and stores, noise control, appropriate lighting, clean air and water, understanding and available safety workers, laws that are equitable and enforced from within (I love the concept of self-policing), and accessible health care and recreation. Comfortable communities are oriented more toward human life and interaction than toward cars, I am certain. These factors have been looked at by community health nursing students as described in the previous chapter. Imagine a community where such assessments and suggestions transform policy.

Watson (2001) describes post-hospital nursing as being different and reconfigured. Nurses will have to know how to gain access to the vast information on the Internet, and pass this information on to their constituents. Then they will facilitate "meaning-making" out of the information obtained. Nurses will be transdisciplinary, in that they can negotiate through the vast array of resources to help clients make choices. Relationships with clients will be intentionally caring, grounded in the community, and will span "birthing, living, aging, changing, growing, and dying" (Watson, 2001, p. 80).

The idea of community comes from the word common—people living together who have in common the same geographical area and share some common values as well. Communities work well when there is general agreement about goals, values, beliefs, and expectations. People have mutual respect for one another and for each others' unique attributes, knowing that these attributes are the spice of life. And there is the conviction that we are all "in this" together—that no man is an island.

This sense of community was brought home to me when my husband and I visited New York City (NYC) a month after the attack. All of our plans had been "cemented" before September 11th and our friend, who had recently moved to NYC, called one week after the attacks to make sure we were still coming. Indeed, he wanted us to come—to help share his angst and receive the comfort of friends, among other things.

Our week in NYC was a poignant reminder to me of the strength of community. We, as tourists, were appreciated, helped, and welcomed. Residents visited with us, taxi drivers talked with us, and restaurant workers shared how their lives had changed as a result of the attack. Crime seemed invisible, to have retreated as if in respect for the heroes and survivors. Individual differences were obscured by the overriding sense that we were all Americans, sharing a national tragedy. The stars and stripes were literally everywhere, and the Statue of Liberty still stood proud in the harbor—these were common symbols and they erased former boundaries. The pain of New Yorkers was our pain; their struggles to rebuild were our struggles. Anxieties about personal safety from further terrorists attacks were acknowledged and experienced and worked through. Most of the activities we had planned to do, we did do, while being fully conscious of the fragility of our safety.

I reflected on my comfort at that time. My comfort need for *relief* from anxiety could not be completely met by anyone. I was never fully at *ease*, but I felt transcendent in post-attack NYC: able to maintain my travel plans in spite of underlying anxiety and psychological pain. I was able to experience *transcendence* because of the palpable sense of community in NYC and the gift of Mayor Guiliani's comforting presence and leadership. The love of America and life in America was expressed universally in Manhattan by persons from all walks of life, all skin colors and languages. Transcendence made all the difference—I came home tired but moved by the power and community of human spirit in NYC. My vision for the 21st century is of human spirits that can be as nurtured and strengthened in all of the communities in which we live and work, as they were in New York.

COMFORT AT THE NATIONAL LEVEL

My mythic vision of comfort at the national level surely has to include some sort of rational (national?) health plan where an identification card provides access to the type of cost-saving community services described above. Political decisions have to be less driven by special interests and campaign finances and more driven by altruistic ideals of equity and unity. Individual rights have to be balanced with mutual respect and regard for fellow Americans and international citizens. National policy has to account for more than our own best interests. Americans must take ownership of policy vision and formulation—we are *all* in this together!

Watson speaks about the nurse as a healing environment. She describes a healing environment as "one that facilitates the emergence of the Haelan effect, the synergistic, organismic multidimensional response of whole persons in the direction of healing and wholeness" (1992, p. 28). Moreover, she directs us to think of the nurse, in addition to being *in* the environment of the client, *as* the environment of the client. Then, we can ask the questions, "If nurses are the environment for the client, how can they be a more healing environment?" and "How can nurses use their consciousness, being, voice, touch, and face for healing?" (1992, p. 27). The idea of a person or group being a healing environment is an interesting idea, and one which was reinforced when I visited the Comfort Diner in NYC.

Comfort Diner Concept

On the first night of our walk around NYC last year, I noticed a bright neon sign that read "Comfort Diner" which had an arrow pointing inside. The colors of this sign were turquoise, red, green, and blue and it was designed in a cheerful, art-deco style. The letters were in very large script—I couldn't miss it. The sign was intentionally nostalgic and welcoming, and the diner itself was converted from a small store that fronted on a main street. It was informal and cozy.

Of course, I had to experience the Comfort Diner and, of course, I loved it! The menu began with the message, "Welcome back to the Golden Age of the diner: Good home cooking, quick service, and popular prices. Enjoy our selection of both classic and new comfort food." The names of the dishes were folksy/traditional as well: Grandma's chicken soup, nice green salad, comfort burger, healthy chicken dish, Thanksgiving everyday, Mom's meatloaf (on her best day), and comforting chicken pie. Truly, these dishes were meant to be comfort food for the soul.

Moreover, the Comfort Diner served many types of ethnic foods: Southern fried chicken, vegetarian chili, comfort quesadillas, and potato pancakes. They served breakfast "anytime" and small plates for children. There were photographs of grandchildren with their grandparents, all happily eating at the diner. Obviously, these messages and the ambience were created very intentionally. And they worked—they conjured up an image of a place where customers feel good and are comforted. Who could resist?

Expanding on these details, I began to experience the diner as a gathering place, rich in social context and common ground. It was oriented to its customers' needs, and was proud of what it could offer and provide. The Comfort Diner had an environment of trust, holism, and tradition, something for everyone with free choice from among familiar and inviting options. There was easy access to the cozy diner, and its booths, stools, tables and chairs seemed dedicated to the customers' comfort. Waiters were cheerful, flexible, and busy and their roles were essential to the missions of the Comfort Diner. (One important mission was to remain profitable.) No request was frowned upon; for example, I purchased two mugs with the Comfort Diner logo on front. It was a place where everyone might "know your name" and care about your comfort, a haven in NYC during these especially stressful times.

My vision for America is that she can become a Comfort Diner for all—where none are excluded, and all feel welcomed and comforted just by being served. I define Comfort Diner as a national human environment that intentionally values and facilitates the comfort and health of its citizens through equity of access, cost, professionalism, caring, technology, support, and respect. The waiters at the diner are analogous to professional and nonprofessional health care providers and care givers, as well as government officials, all of whom are themselves healing environments. America would thus be dedicated to the comfort and health of all of its citizens. Where relief and ease aren't fully possible, transcendence is facilitated by leaders who instill hope instead of despair, strength instead of powerlessness, support instead of isolation. When cure isn't possible, Americans are supported in making choices that assure their dignity and the honoring of their health care desires. They are supported in reaching a new kind of healing.

COMFORT AT THE GLOBAL LEVEL

If America is a Comfort Diner, then the nations of the world could be too. Picture these Diners* as unique human environments, lined up on 5th Avenue, serving whoever walks in their doors. While each Diner identifies with a national origin, each is inclusive of anyone who wants to sample the menu. The Diners share successful business strategies and no one Diner believes it is more important than another. Each is respectful of the uniqueness and strengths of the others. Some Diners may have more experience or are larger than others, and those Diners serve as models and helpers for the others. They share staff and supplies

---

*In this mythic vision, Diner (capitalized) refers to the restaurant, not a person *in* the restaurant.

when necessary, communicating through a Comfort Diners' Association. Rules for doing business on 5th Avenue are voted upon by representatives to the Association from all of the Diners, who are chosen freely by the customers, waiters, and managers. Also, each Diner contributes, in proportion to its income, to a 5th Avenue fund which is used for emergencies such as natural disasters and fires.

The vitality of 5th Avenue is dependent upon all of the Diners cooperating, being mindful of the cleanliness and safety of their avenue and their mission of serving and comforting everyone. They help those customers who are unable to come to 5th Avenue. Each Diner is free to choose its management style and each Diner is self-governed and self-policed . . . I could go on and on. It is a fun metaphor to play with and envision. Just pondering such a vision in a book such as this is a step toward questioning whether human living can be more harmonious and value-centered than it presently is.

The image of Comfort Diners lined up with their own colorful signs written in their own languages is a fanciful one: Conforto da Pranzo (Italy), Confortar Comensal (Spain), Ytewenne Pectopah (Russian), Dineur a Confort (French), Utecha Jidelna (Czech), Komfort Speisewagen (German), et cetera. This 5th Avenue image helps illustrate that the term, comfort, seems to be quite universal—at least comfort is present in the translation resources that I had available. (In addition to these Indo European countries, I have had inquiries about Comfort Theory from nurses in Norway, Portugal, Thailand, China, Turkey, and Sri Lanka.) This leads me to believe that comfort in any language refers to essentially the same gestalt, at least in patient care.

I believe that comfort is a concept that binds us together globally as nurses and as an integral part of wider health care delivery systems. Comfort as a scientific term was first explored in nursing, but all fruits of this exploration point to it being an interdisciplinary concept. Thus, comfort is useful for all disciplines as a unifying *framework* for designing interventions, working toward realistic goals that patients and families want and will work to achieve. It has been postulated here that when nurses and other members of the team use the framework of Comfort Care, their health care institutions will become stronger. Think of how these effects can be enlarged when more health care professionals around the world do something about the health care needs of persons not able to come to clinics and hospitals. Opportunities abound in organizations like HOPE (Helping Other People Everywhere) Healthcorp run by the International Churches of Christ (Pohlkotte, 2001).

Transcultural Comfort

Much work is needed to translate Comfort Theory, and this book, into other languages so that comfort, as a measurable outcome for health care, becomes explicit and valued. On the other hand, it is possible that the World Wide Web will facilitate translations, as there are programs on the Web that enable most Web pages to be converted into specified languages. As more and more countries with their native languages participate in such Internet programs, perhaps The Comfort Line (Kolcaba, K., 1997) will be utilized in a variety of cultures.

Health

The World Health Organization (WHO) formulated a classic definition of health as "a state of complete physical, mental, and social well-being and not merely the absence of disease or infirmity" (1974, p. 1). Pender (1996) pointed out that not only is health multidimensional but applicable to aggregates as well as individuals. Health is a dynamic process inherent in the life experience of families, communities, and nations.

On my Web pages in the FAQ section, I define health as optimum function of a patient/family/community facilitated by enhanced comfort (Kolcaba, K., 1997). Comfort theory states that enhanced comfort is related to engagement by the patient, family, or community in HSBs. Thus health is an active, participatory process. We know that we have to work to maintain our health, and we have to work to maintain healthy communities, nations, and our planet. We each have a role to play, starting with other-directed commitments to enhance comfort in our spheres of influence.

Peace

One of my favorite old hymns talks about peace thusly:

> Let there be peace on earth, and let it begin with me.
> Let there be peace on earth, the peace that was meant to be.

I noticed as I sang it again, though, that the hymn doesn't tell us *how* to walk in "perfect harmony." I would suggest that, in addition to working on our own peaceful feelings, we can also help along the cause of peace by being aware of the comfort of others. It is not enough anymore to promote only our individual freedoms and rights; we must work toward the freedoms, rights, and comfort of others. Our perspective can start with contemplating and addressing comfort needs inherent in humankind. A perspective that is other-directed precludes greed and advocates for equity. Many individuals already practice such a life. Can we say the same for our corporations and nations?

We can remember, however, that corporations and nations are made up of individuals and stockholders. Individuals can make their values known. We can become a more peaceful planet, inch by inch, and comfort measure by comfort measure. If comfort of others is a value that we agree upon, let us then be committed to spreading comfort to those around us.

The Nature of Peace

Peace is not the product of terror or fear.
Peace is not the silence of cemeteries.
Peace is not the result of violent repression.
Peace is the generous, tranquil contribution of all to the good of all.
Peace is dynamism. Peace is generosity. It is right and duty.

—Archbishop Oscar Romero, 1984, "The Church Is All of You"

COMFORT WORK FOR THE FUTURE

Using ourselves as instruments of comfort, we can volunteer in our congregations and communities. We can address comfort needs in our small worlds; if enough of us do this, our circles of comfort will begin to intersect and grow larger. We can advocate for other circles, other Comfort Diners, showing by example how "peace is the generous, tranquil contribution of all to the good of all" (Archbishop Romero). Peace must be other-directed and intentional, and it can be facilitated by thinking about the holistic comfort needs of others. As actor Martin Sheen stated recently, "I've protested, calling attention to my country's dark spots, because I love America so much. I learned that, to keep your life from becoming self-contained and useless, you have to feel other people's pain and act to help them. That is what faith and love are all about" (interview with D. Rader, 2001).

In a less altruistic, but equally important vein, comfort of others will be valued more by our capitalistic society if we demonstrate how this approach has concrete benefits for institutions, agencies, and governments. Table 10.1 presents a realistic set of priorities, as I see the quest, for promoting Comfort Care in the 21st century. If you and/or your colleagues are working in any of these areas or others that are not listed, please publish your positive *or* negative findings. It is also important to add your publications or others that you find useful to The Comfort Line (by contacting me) so that new knowledge can be integrated into present knowledge. I would also appreciate your communications and questions—I learn much from your feedback.

TABLE 10.1   Future Directions for Comfort Care

Practice	Adopt Comfort Care as framework for practice on individual units; adapt it for practice setting; implement bottom-up management model. You can try this as an interdisciplinary model, such as an ACE unit, or as a nursing model.
	Clinical ladder research about interventions that enhance comfort.
	Clinical ladder research to show how comfort is related HSBs and Institutional Outcomes.
	Lobby for magnet designation for your health care organization (American Nurses Association, 2001).
Education	Teach students at all levels the art of Comfort Care.
	Ask students to complete patient and patient/family care plans (see Figures 10.1 and 10.2) for their own patients or clients in different settings.
	Present model in Continuing Education classes to staff nurses and other disciplines.
	Participate in transcultural nursing experiences (Pohlkotte, 2001).
Research	Starting with small pilot studies, demonstrate cost effectiveness of Comfort Care compared with units that do not use the framework.
	Conduct field research about interventions that enhance comfort.
	Conduct field research to show how comfort is related to HSBs and Institutional Outcomes.
	Translate General Comfort Questionnaire into other languages and test psychometric properties (reliability and validity) of those instruments.
	Utilize on common database for research (for example, NIC/NOC) (Iowa Intervention Project, 1996; Iowa Outcomes Project, 1997).
	Think about and develop norms for comfort cutoff scores, below which action would be triggered.
	Measure comfort in children, developmentally disabled adults, and other unique populations.

Patient _____ Medical Diagnosis _____ Nurse/Student _____

Comfort Needs	Interventions	Intervening Variables	Patient's Perception Of Own Comfort	What Next?	Health Seeking Behaviors	Institutional Outcomes
	The Nurse will…				*The patient will…*	
Physical			Objective			
Psychospiritual			Subjective		Internal and/or	
Environmental					External and/or	
Sociocultural			Supporting		Peaceful Death	

FIGURE 10.1 Patient Comfort Care plan.

Caregiver/Family Nurse/Student		Patient			Medical Diagnosis			
Comfort Needs of Family	Comfort Needs of Patient	Interventions	Intervening Variables	Patient's Perception of Own Comfort	Family's Perception of Their Comfort	What Next?	Health Seeking Behaviors	Institutional Outcomes
Physical	Physical	*The Nurse will…*		Objective	Objective		*The patient/family will…*	
Psychospiritual	Psychospiritual			Subjective	Subjective		Internal Behaviors	
Sociocultural	Sociocultural			Supporting	Supporting		External Behaviors	
Environmental	Environmental						Peaceful Death	

FIGURE 10.2   Family/patient Comfort Care plan.

201

Because patient comfort is so complex, many building blocks are yet to be discovered and placed within the structure of health care knowledge (Kolcaba & Wykle, 1997). To add details to this structure will take the interest, skills, and cooperation of many. So, come into our Comfort Circle or start your own and help our circles grow together!

MUSINGS ON COMFORT QUOTES (CHAPTER 10)

> Across the nation Friday [September 14, 2001], people gathered to comfort each other during a national day of prayer. . . . Participants joined hands for a moment of silence.
>
> —Brazaitis, T., "The survivors need help too."
> *Cleveland Plain Dealer*, September 16, 2001, p. H-3

This quote demonstrates the commonality of comfort—the innate tendency to seek out other persons when we need comfort. The quote shows how, when we acknowledge and act on our common needs for comfort, we somehow receive comfort from those we are comforting. I have found this to be the case in our hand massage research with hospice patients: I come away from those massage sessions strengthened and inspired! So ministering to the comfort needs of others is another win-win proposition.

> We said I love you a thousand times over and over again, and it just brought so much peace to us," says Lyz [wife of Jeremy Glick, hero on Flight 93 out of Newark, which crashed in Pennsylvania on September 11, 2001]. "I felt the feeling from it. He told me, "I love Emmy"—who is our daughter—"and to take care of her." Then he said, "Whatever decisions you make in your life, I need you to be happy, and I will respect any decisions that you make." That's what he said and that gives me the most comfort. He sounded strong. He didn't sound panicked, very clear-headed. I told him to put a picture of me and Emmy in his head to be strong. . . . And then he said, "I need some advice . . . we're talking about attacking these men, what

should I do?" And then I finally just decided at that instant that "Honey, you need to do it."
—Elyzabeth Glick (wife of Jeremy Glick) interviewed by Jane Pauley on Dateline, NBC, September 18, 2001

This heartfelt quote reflects the importance of respect when comforting others. When people need comfort, they also need respect. We are vulnerable when we have needs for comfort and would-be comforters must convey their reverence for those in need. Comforting should be unconditional as well. These aspects are, after all, part of the strengthening power of comfort.

"I think about the families, the children," the president told reporters gathered in the Oval Office, looking away for a moment to compose himself. "I wish I could comfort every single family whose lives have been affected."
—George W. Bush, as reported by Bob Kemper, *Chicago Tribune*, September 14, 2001, pp. 1–3

The third quote speaks to the instinctive human capacity and desire to comfort others, when we are in the position to do so. We can maximize this capacity as we create our own comfort circles and Comfort Diners. We can speak about comfort as a resurrected value for health care and living in the 21st century.

Dzemila Spahovic is a case manager with the refugee mental health program reporting about her nightmares Tuesday night, after the attack on America. "When I came here, I hoped we would stay safe for all time," she said as she is counseling Bosnians who are confused, unable to sleep, and afraid of sudden noises. Spahovic said it can be difficult to offer comfort while haunted by her own fears. "But," she said, smiling. "Somebody has to do it."
—Dzemila Spahovic, as reported by J. Lieblich and S. Franklin, *Chicago Tribune*, September 14, 2001, pp. 1–11

Please remember, we all know that it can be difficult to offer comfort in the midst of our own family responsibilities and fatigue. But, "*somebody has to do it*" and all those somebodies add up to power, to ever-widening comfort circles, to Comfort Diners, and to a 5th Avenue lined with international Comfort Diners. Please join us and become part of our Comfort Team! We need you.

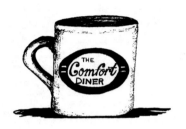

References

Aikens, C. (1908). Making the patient comfortable. *Canadian Nurse and Hospital Review, 4*(9), 422–424.

Ambuel, B., Hamlett, K., Marx, C., & Blumer, J. (1992). Assessing distress in pediatric intensive care environments: The COMFORT scale. *Journal of Pediatric Psychology, 17*(1), 95–109.

American Nurses Association. (1991). *Position statement for promotion of comfort and relief of pain in dying patients.* Washington, DC: Author.

American Nurses Association. (1994). *Position statement against assisted suicide* Washington, DC: Author.

American Nurses Association. (2001). Mandatory overtime bill caps off successful legislative year. *The American Nurse, 33*(6), 3, 17.

American Nurses Association and Health Ministries Association, Inc. (1998). *Scope and standards of parish nursing practice.* New York: American Nurses Association Publishing.

Andrews, C., & Chrzanowski, M. (1990). Maternal position, labor, and comfort. *Applied Nursing Research, 3*(1), 7–13.

Arrington, D., & Walborn, K. (1989). The comfort caregiver concept. *Caring, 8*(12), 24–27.

Benner, P. (1984). *From novice to expert.* Reading, MA: Addison-Wesley Publishing Co.

Berry, T. (1988). *The dream of the earth.* San Francisco: Sierra Club Books.

Bishop, S. (1998). Logical reasoning. In A. Tomey & M. Alligood (Eds.), *Nursing theorists and their work* (pp. 25–34). St. Louis, MO: Mosby.

Blum, L. (1992). Care. In L. Becker & C. Becker (Eds.), *Encyclopedia of ethics* (Vol. I, A-K; pp. 125–126). New York: Garland Publishing Co.

Buerhaus, P., & Needleman, J. (2000). Policy implication of research on nurse staffing and quality of care. *Policy, Politics, & Nursing Practice, 1*, 5–16.

Buerhaus, P., & Norman, L. (2001). It's time to require theory and methods of quality improvement in basic and graduate nursing education. *Nursing Outlook, 49*, 67–69.

Burns, R. (1838). The tree of liberty. In W. Henley & T. Henderson (Eds.), *The poetry of Robert Burns*. Scotland: Edinburgh Press.

Brazaitis, T. (2001). September 16, p. H-3. The survivors need help too. The Plain Dealer (Cleveland, OH).

Carpenito, L. (1987). *Nursing diagnosis: Application to clinical practice*. Philadelphia: J. B. Lippincott.

Chinn, P. (1992). From the editor. *Advances in Nursing Science, 15*(1), vii.

Coile, Z. (2001, Sept. 23). "Giuliani gains popularity in the aftermath of tragedy." *The Plain Dealer*. Cleveland, OH, p. A9.

Cook, J. (2000). Caregiver's Comfort. Caregivers' Comfort Creations, LLC, P.O. Box 6323. Evanston, IL 60204.

Council of Nurses. (1973). Center for Study of Ethics in the Professions [On-line]. International Council of Nurses, Code for Nurses. http://csep.iit.edu/Codes/coe/International.

Cox, J. (1996). Assessing patient comfort in radiation therapy. *Radiation Therapist, 5*(2), 119–125.

Craik, D. (1969). *Friendship*. Norwalk, CT: C. R. Gibson Co.

Daily Word. (2001). Presence. *Daily Word,* July, p. 45.

Derman, M., & Huber, D. (1999). Patient outcomes: A measure of nursing's value. *American Journal of Nursing, 99*(9), 40–48.

Donahue, M. P. (1989). *Nursing: The finest art*. St. Louis: Mosby.

Dowd, T. (2001). Katharine Kolcaba: Theory of Comfort Theory. In A. Tomey & M. Alligood (Eds.), *Nursing theorists and their work* (5th ed., pp. 430–442). St. Louis: Mosby.

Dowd, T., & Dowd, E. T. (1995). Cognitive therapy in the management of urinary incontinence. *Complessita & Cambiamento (Complexity and Change), 4*(2), 11–15.

Dowd, T., Kolcaba, K., & Steiner, R. (2000). Using cognitive strategies to enhance bladder control and comfort. *Holistic Nursing Practice, 14*(2), 91–103.

Dowd, T., Kolcaba, K., & Steiner, R. (2002). Correlations among measures of bladder function and comfort. *Journal of Nursing Measurement, 10*(1), 27–38.

Downing, J. C. (2000). *Caregivers' Comfort Creations, LLC*. P.O. Box 6323, Evanston, IL, 60204.

Dozor, R., & Addison, R. (1992). Toward a good death: An interpretive investigation of family practice residents' practices with dying patients. *Family Medicine, 24*, 538–543.

Dretske, F. (1988). *Explaining behavior: Reasons in a world of causes*. Cambridge, MA: MIT Press.

Family Circle. (2001). Comfort is the key to looking good. August, p. 73.

Fawcett, J. (1984). The metaparadigm of nursing: Present status and future refinements. *Image: The Journal of Nursing Scholarship, 16*(2), 84–89.

Ferguson, V. (1989). The nurse executive: Comfort and presence. *Journal of Professional Nursing, 5*(6), 289.

Foley, M. (2001). Staffing: The ANA's primary concern. *American Journal of Nursing, 101*(1), 88.

Fortin, J. (1999). Human needs and nursing theory. In H. Kim & I. Kollak (Eds.), *Nursing theories: Conceptual and philosophical foundations* (pp. 23–54). New York: Springer Publishing.

Fox, C., & Kolcaba, K. (1995). Unsafe practice: A lack of strategies for effective decision making. (News, notes, and tips). *Nurse Educator, 20*(5), 3–4.

Fuller, S. (1978). Holistic man and the science of nursing. *Nursing Outlook, 26,* 700–704.

Funk, S., Tornquist, E., Champagne, M., Copp, L., & Wiese, R. (1989). *Key aspects of comfort: Management of pain, fatigue, and nausea.* New York: Springer Publishing.

Glaser, C., & Strauss, A. (1965). *Awareness of dying.* Chicago: Aldine.

Goodnow, M. (1935). *The technic of nursing.* Philadelphia: W. B. Saunders.

Goodwin, L., & Goodwin, W. (1991). Focus on psychometrics: Estimating construct validity. *Research in Nursing and Health, 14,* 235–243.

Gropper, E. (1992). Promoting health by promoting comfort. *Nursing Forum, 27*(2), 5–8.

Halloway, T. (2001). A day in the life of a nurse. *Registered Nursing, 64*(7), 54.

Hamilton, J. (1989). Comfort and the hospitalized chronically ill. *Journal of Gerontological Nursing, 15*(4), 28–33.

Harmer, B. (1926). *Methods and principles of teaching the principles and practice of nursing.* New York: MacMillan.

Harmer, B. (1931). *Textbook of the principles and practice of nursing* (2nd ed.). New York: MacMillan.

Health Information Policy Council. (1985). 1984 revision of the uniform hospital discharge data set. *Federal Register, 50*(147), 31038–31040.

Henderson, V. (1978). *Principles and practice of nursing.* New York: Macmillan.

Hinds, P. (1984). Inducing a definition of "hope" through the use of grounded theory methodology. *Journal of Advanced Nursing, 9,* 357–362.

Hogan-Miller, E., Rustad, D., Sendelbach, S., & Goldenberg, I. (1995). Effects of three methods of femoral site immobilization on bleeding and comfort after coronary angiogram. *American Journal of Critical Care, 4*(2), 143–148.

Howarth, F. (1982). A holistic view of middle management. *Nursing Outlook, 30,* 522–552.

HRSA (2001, April 20). HHS study finds strong link between patient outcomes and nurse staffing in hospitals. *Health Resources and Services Administration Report* [On-line]. http://www.hrsa.gov/Newsroom/releases/2001%20Releases/nursestudy.htm/.

Humphreys, G. (1989). Dear nurse. *American Journal of Nursing*, Nov.

Hurley, A., Volicer, B., Hanrahan, S., & Volicer, L. (1992). Assessment of discomfort in advanced Alzheimer patient. *Research in Nursing & Health*, *15*, 369–377.

International Council of Nurses (ICN), Geneva. (2000). *Code for nurses.* Geneva: Imprimeries Populaires. Online: http://www.icn.ch/icncode.pdf

International Parish Nurse Resource Center. (1999). On-line: www.advocatehealth.com/sites/pnursctr.html/.

Iowa Intervention Project. (1996). *Nursing interventions classification (NOC)* (J. McCloskey & G. Bulechek, Eds., 2nd ed.). St. Louis: Mosby.

Iowa Outcomes Project. (1997). *Nursing outcomes classification (NOC)* (M. Johnson & M. Maas, Eds.). St. Louis: Mosby.

Jenkins, G., & Taber, T. (1977). A Monte Carlo study of factors affecting three indices of composite scale reliability. *Journal of Applied Psychology*, *62*, 392–398.

Jennings, B., Staggers, N., & Brosch, L. (1999). A classification scheme for outcome indicators. *Image: Journal of Nursing Scholarship, 31*(4), 381–388.

Johnson, M., & Maas, M. (1999). Nursing-sensitive patient outcomes. In E. Cohen & V. DeBack (Eds.), *The outcomes mandate* (pp. 37–48). St. Louis: Mosby.

Johnson, S. (1750). The Rambler #21. In *A Johnson Reader.* New York: Pantheon Books, 1964, p. 172.

Karnofsky, D., & Burchenal, J. (1949). The clinical evaluation of chemotherapeutic agents against cancer. In N. McLeod (Ed.), *Evaluation of chemotherapeutic agents* (pp. 191–205). New York: Columbia University Press.

Keeling, A., Knight, E., Taylor, V., & Nordt, L. (1994). Postcardiac catheterization time-in-bed study: Enhancing patient comfort through nursing research. *Applied Nursing Research, 7*(1), 14–17.

Kemper, B. (2001). "I wish I could comfort every . . . " President Bush quote, *Chicago Tribune*, pp. 1–3.

Kendall, G., Hrycaiko, D., & Martino, G. (1990). The effects of an imagery rehearsal, relaxation, and self-talk package on basketball game performance. *Journal of Sport and Exercise Psychology, 12*, 157–166.

Kim, H. (1999). Introduction. In H. Kim & I. Kollak (Eds.), *Nursing theories: Conceptual and philosophical foundations* (pp. 1–7). New York: Springer Publishing.

Knapp, T., Kimble, L., & Dunbar, S. (1998). Distinguishing between the stability of a construct and the stability of an instrument in trait/state measurement. *Nursing Research, 47,* 60–61.

Koff, S. (2001, Jan. 21). He calls for building character, banishing hidden prejudices. *The Plain Dealer.* Cleveland, OH, p. A1.

Kolcaba, K. (1987). Reaching optimum function is realistic goal for elderly. (Letter to the Editor). *Journal of Gerontological Nursing, 13*(12), 36.

Kolcaba, K. (1988). A framework for the nursing care of demented patients. *Mainlines, 9*(6), 12–13.

Kolcaba, K. (1991). A taxonomic structure for the concept comfort. *Image: Journal of Nursing Scholarship, 23*(4), 237–239.

Kolcaba, K. (1992a). The concept of comfort in an environmental framework. *Journal of Gerontological Nursing, 18*(6), 33–38.

Kolcaba, K. (1992b). Holistic comfort: Operationalizing the construct as a nurse-sensitive outcome. *Advances in Nursing Science, 15*(1), 1–10.

Kolcaba, K. (1994). A theory of holistic comfort for nursing. *Journal of Advanced Nursing, 19,* 1178–1184.

Kolcaba, K. (1994, October). "Give Us Better Advice." Letter to the editor. *The American Nurse.*

Kolcaba, K. (1995a). The process and product of comfort merged in holistic nursing art. *Journal of Holistic Nursing Practice, 13*(2), 117–131.

Kolcaba, K. (1995b). The art of comfort care. *Image: Journal of Nursing Scholarship, 27*(4), 287–289.

Kolcaba, K. (1997). *The Comfort Line* [On-line]. Available: http://www.uakron.edu/comfort/.

Kolcaba, K. (1998). The effects of guided imagery on comfort in women with breast cancer choosing conservative therapy. (Doctoral dissertation, Case Western Reserve University, 1997). *Dissertation Abstracts International,* DAI-B 58/07. Jan. p. 3558.

Kolcaba, K. (1998). Comfort. *The encyclopedia of nursing research* (pp. 102–104). New York: Springer Publishing.

Kolcaba, K. (1998, May). The art of comfort care. *Summa Research Progress Newsletter.*

Kolcaba, K. (1999, Sept.). Guided imagery study cited in *American Health Magazine,* p. 47.

Kolcaba, K. (2000). Holistic care: Is it feasible in today's health care environment? [Counterpoint Response]. *Nursing Leadership Forum, 4*(4), 105–107. [Reprinted in *Nursing leaders speak out: Issues and opinions* (pp. 49–54). (2001). New York: Springer Publishing.]

Kolcaba, K. (2001). Evolution of the mid-range theory of comfort for outcomes research. *Nursing Outlook, 49*(2), 86–92.

Kolcaba, K. (2001). Kolcaba's Theory of Comfort. *Core concepts for advanced nursing practice* (pp. 418–422). St. Louis: Mosby.

Kolcaba, K. (in review). The Theory of Comfort. Chapter in *Middle Range Theories: Application to Nursing Research.* New York: Lippincott, Williams, & Wilkins.

Kolcaba, K., & Dowd, T. (2000). Kegel exercises: Strengthening the weak pelvic floor muscles that cause urinary incontinence. *American Journal of Nursing, 100*(11), 59.

Kolcaba, K., & Fisher, E. (1996). A holistic perspective on comfort care as an advance directive. *Critical Care Nursing Quarterly, 18*(4), 66–76.

Kolcaba, K., & Fox, C. (1999). The effects of guided imagery on comfort of women with early stage breast cancer undergoing radiation therapy. *Oncology Nursing Forum, 26*(1), 67–72.

Kolcaba, K., & Kolcaba, R. (1991). An analysis of the concept of comfort. *Journal of Advanced Nursing, 16,* 1301–1310.

Kolcaba, K., & Steiner, R. (2000). Empirical evidence for the nature of holistic comfort. *Journal of Holistic Nursing, 18*(1), 46–62.

Kolcaba, K., & Wilson, L. (2002). Comfort Care: A framework for Peri-Anesthesia nursing. *Journal of PeriAnesthesia Nursing, 17*(2), 102–114.

Kolcaba, K., & Wykle, M. (1997). Spreading comfort around the world. *Reflections,* 2nd quarter, 12–13.

Kolcaba, R. (1997). The primary holisms in nursing. *Journal of Advanced Nursing, 25,* 290–296.

Kovner, C., Harrington, C., & Mezey, M. (2001). Counting nurses: What is community health-public health nursing? *American Journal of Nursing, 101*(1), 59–60.

Kozier, B., Erb, G., Berman, A., & Burke, K. (2000). Caring, comforting, and communicating. *Fundamentals of nursing: Concepts, process, and practice* (6th ed., pp. 430–431). New York: Prentice Hall.

Krueger, B. (2001, June 16). Dear Abby. *The Plain Dealer,* p. 10-E.

Labun, E. (1988). Spiritual care: An element in nursing care planning. *Journal of Advanced Nursing, 13,* 314–320.

Landefeld, S., Palmer, R., Kresevic, D., Fortinsky, R., & Kowal, J. (1995). A randomized trail of care in a hospital medical unit especially designed to improve the functional outcomes of acutely ill older patients. *New England Journal of Medicine, 332*(29), 1338–1344.

Laurie, R. (2001, July 1). "We must educate . . . " Letter to the editor: Do doctors owe patients optimism, or the truth? *The Plain Dealer,* p. 4-G.

Lee, C. (1990). Psyching up for a muscular endurance task: Effects of image content on performance and mood state. *Journal of Sport and Exercise Psychology, 12,* 66–73.

Lehman, D. (2001, July 22). *Jacobs Field, Game Face.* Dennis Lehman, Indians VP of Business, p. 24.

Levine, M. (1967). The four conservation principles of nursing. *Nursing Forum, 6,* 45–49.

Lieblick, J., & Franklin, S. (2001, Sept. 14). "Somebody has to do it." Article "Refugees relive homeland terror, comfort U.S. natives." *Chicago Tribune.* Section 1, p. 11.

Lipsey, M. (1990). *Design sensitivity.* Newbury Park, CA: Sage.

Louden, J. (1992). *The woman's comfort book.* San Francisco: Harper.

Lynn, M. (1986). Determination and quantification of content validity. *Nursing Research, 35,* 352–385.

Mallison, M. (1990). Editorial. *American Journal of Nursing* (Oct.), p. 15.

Malone, B. N. (1999). All I want for Christmas. *The American Nurse* (Nov./Dec.), p. 4.

McClelland, D. (1988). The effect of motivational arousal through films on salivary immunoglobulin A. *Psychological Health, 2,* 31–52.

McIlveen, K., & Morse, J. (1995). The role of comfort in nursing care: 1900–1980. *Clinical Nursing Research, 4*(2), 127–148.

Melzak, R., & Wall, P. (1982). *The challenge of pain.* New York: Basic Books.

MetroHealth System. (1999). *Pain management: Comfort with caring* [Brochure #44109-1998]. Cleveland, OH: Author.

Miller, C. (1999). (Contributor, Chapters 1, 2, 22). *Nursing care of older adults* (3rd ed.). New York: J. B. Lippincott.

Morse, J. (1983). An ethnoscientific analysis of comfort: A preliminary investigation. *Nursing Papers, 15,* 6–20.

Morse, J. (1992). Comfort: The refocusing of nursing care. *Clinical Nursing Research, 1*(1), 91–106.

Murray, H. (1938). *Explorations in personality.* New York: Oxford Press.

National Committee on Vital and Health Statistics. (1980). *Long-term health care: Minimum data set* (No. PHS 80-1158). Washington, DC: U.S. Department of Health and Human Services.

National Committee on Vital and Health Statistics. (1981). *Uniform ambulatory medical care: Minimum data set* (No. PHS 81-1161). Washington, DC: U.S. Department of Health and Human Services.

National Hospice Organization. (1994). Standards of a hospice program of care. *The Hospice Journal, 9*(4), 39–74.

Neves-Arruda, E., Larson, P., & Meleis, A. (1992). Comfort: Immigrant Hispanic cancer patients' views. *Cancer Nursing, 15*(6), 387–394.

Nightingale, F. (1859). *Notes on nursing.* London: Harrison.

Nolan, M., & Grant, G. (1992). Mid-range theory building and the nursing theory-practice gap: A respite care case study. *Journal of Advanced Nursing, 17,* 217–223.

Novak, B., Kolcaba, K., Steiner, R., & Dowd, T. (2001). Measuring comfort in caregivers and patients during late end-of-life care. *American Journal of Hospice & Palliative Care, 18*(3), 170–180.

Nowotny, M. (1989). Assessment of hope in patients with cancer: Development of an instrument. *Oncology Nursing Forum, 16*(1), 57–61.

Nursing Outcomes Classification. (2000). M. Johnson, M. Maas, & S. Moorhead (Eds.), 2nd Ed. St. Louis: Mosby.

Oaster, T. (1989). Number of alternative per choice point and stability of Likert-type scales. *Perceptual and Motor Skills, 68,* 549–550.

Oerlemans, M. (1972). Eli. *American Journal of Nursing, 72,* 1440–1441.

Orlando, I. (1961/1990). *The dynamic nurse-patient relationship.* New York: National League for Nursing.

Orr, R., Paris, J., & Siegler, M. (1991). Caring for the terminally ill: Resolving conflicting objectives between patient, physician, family, and institution. *Journal of Family Practice, 33,* 500–504.

Palmer, R., Landefeld, S., Kresevic, D., & Kowal, J. (1994). A medical unit for the acute care of the elderly. *Journal of the American Geriatric Society, 42*(5), 545–552.

Panno, J., Kolcaba, K., & Holder, C. (2000). Acute Care for Elders (ACE): A holistic model for geriatric orthopaedic nursing care. *Orthopaedic Nursing, 19*(6), 1–9.

Paterson, J., & Zderad, L. (1976/1988). *Humanistic nursing.* New York: National League for Nursing.

Pender, N. (1996). *Health promotion in nursing practice* (3rd ed.). Stamford, CT: Appleton & Lange.

Peplau, H. (1952). The art and science of nursing: Similarities, differences, and relations. *Nursing Science Quarterly, 1*(1), 5–15.

Phillips, L., & Ayres, M. (1999). Supportive and nonsupportive care environments for the elderly. In A. Hinshaw, S. Feetham, & J. Shaver (Eds.), *Handbook of clinical nursing research* (pp. 600–603). Thousand Oaks, CA: Sage.

Pohlkotte, A. (2001). The ultimate nursing adventure: Student discovers a passion for transcultural nursing. *Excellence in clinical practice, 4th quarter, 2*(4), 1–4. (Published by Sigma Theta Tau International.)

Rader, D. (2001, Dec. 2). I discovered what faith and love are really about. *Parade Magazine, The Sunday Newspaper Magazine* (pp. 4–6). New York: Parade Publications.

Rankin-Box, D. (1986). Comfort. *Nursing (London): The Journal of Clinical Practice, Education, and Management, 3*(9), 340–342.

Rasmussen, J. (1989). Analysis of Likert-scale data: A reinterpretation of Gregoire and Driver. *Psychological Bulletin, 105* 167–170.

Reed, P. (1987). Spirituality and well-being in terminally ill hospitalized adults. *Research in Nursing and Health, 10,* 335–344.

Robinson, D., & Kish, C. (2001). Core Concepts in Advanced Practice Nursing. Section VI, Theoretical Foundations. *Kolcaba's Theory of Comfort,* pp. 418–422. St. Louis: Mosby.

Robinson, E. (2001). Ethical issues: Caring for incompetent patients and their surrogates. *American Journal of Nursing, 101*(7), 75–76.

Romero, O. (1984). The church is all of you. In J. Brockman (Ed.), *The nature of peace* (p. 24). Minneapolis, MN: Winston Press.

Roy, C., & Roberts, S. (1981). *Theory construction in nursing: An adaptation model.* Englewood Cliffs, NJ: Prentice Hall.

Saltus, R. (2001, April 27). Number of nurses affects patient health. *Cleveland Plain Dealer, Health Section.*

Schlotfeldt, R. (1975). The need for a conceptual framework. In P. Verhonic (Ed.), *Nursing research* (pp. 3–25). Boston: Little & Brown.

Schoener, C., & Krysan, L. (1996). The comfort and discomfort of infertility. *JOGNN, 25*(2), 167–172.

Schuiling, K., & Sampselle, C. (1999). Comfort in labor and midwifery art. *Image: Journal of Nursing Scholarship, 31*(1), 77–81.

Schwab, M., Rader, J., & Doan, J. (1985). Relieving the anxiety and fear in dementia. *Journal of Gerontological Nursing, 11*(5), 8–15.

Shakespeare, W. (~1598). King Henry the Fifth. Act II. Scene III. In P. Alexander (Ed.), *The complete works of Shakespeare* (p. 561). London: Collins.

Shrout, P., & Fleiss, J. (1979). Intraclass correlations: Uses in assessing rater reliability. *Psychological Bulletin, 86,* 420–428.

Simon, E. (1999, Dec. 3). Bottom-up management no longer on the fringe. *The Plain Dealer,* p. 3-H.

Spielberger, C. (1983). *Manual for the State-Trait Anxiety Inventory.* Palo Alto, CA: Consulting Psychologists Press, Inc.

Stegner, W. (1988). *Crossing to safety.* New York: Penguin Books.

Stevens, J. (1992). *Applied multivariate statistics for the social sciences* (2nd ed.). Hillsdale, NJ: Lawrence Erlbaum Associates.

Suin, R. (1972). Removing emotional obstacles to learning and performance by visuo-motor behavior rehearsal. *Behavior Therapy, 3U,* 308–310.

Tabachnick, B., & Fidell, L. (1989). *Using multivariate statistics* (2nd ed.). New York: Harper & Row.

Tomey, A., & Alligood, M. (Eds.). (2001). *Nursing theorists and their work* (5th ed.). St. Louis: Mosby.

United Nations. (2000). *The universal declaration of human rights.* New York: Author.

U.S. Department of Health and Human Services. (2000). *Healthy people 2010: Understanding and improving health* (2nd ed.). Washington, DC: U.S. Government Printing Office. Also on-line at http://www.health.gov/healthypeople/.

Van Dijk, M., De Boer, J., Koot, H., Tibboel, D., Passchier, J., & Duivenvoorden, H. (2000). The reliability and validity of the comfort scale as a postoperative pain instrument in 0–3-year-old infants. *Pain, 84*(2–3), 367–377.

Vendlinski, S., & Kolcaba, K. (1997). Comfort care: A framework for hospice nursing. *The American Journal of Hospice & Palliative Care, 14*(6), 1–6.

Vullo-Navich, K., Smith, S., Andrews, M., Levine, A., Tischler, J., & Veglis, J. (1998). Comfort and incidence of abnormal serum sodium, BUN, creatinine and osmolality in dehydration of terminal illness. *The American Journal of Hospice & Palliative Care, 15*(2), 77–84.

Walker, L., & Avant, K. (1988). *Strategies for theory construction in nursing* (2nd ed.). Norwalk, CT: Appleton & Lange.

Walker, L., & Avant, K. (1995). *Strategies for theory construction in nursing* (3rd ed.). Norwalk, CT: Appleton & Lange.

Watson, J. (1979). *Nursing: The philosophy and science of caring.* Boulder, CO: Colorado Associated University Press.

Watson, J. (1992). Holding sacred space: The nurse as healing environment. *Holistic Nursing Practice, 6*(4), 26–36.

Watson, J. (2001). Post-hospital nursing: Shortage, shifts, and scripts. *Nursing Administration Quarterly, 25*(3), 77–82.

Webster's New Universal Unabridged Dictionary. (1979). Deluxe Second Edition. J. McHechne (Editor). New York: Simon & Shuster.

Webster's New World Dictionary. (1995). V. Neufeldt & A. Sparks (Eds.). New York: Simon & Schuster, Pocket Books Division.

Westberg, G. (1990). *The parish nurse: Providing a minister of health for your congregation.* Minneapolis: Augsburg Press.

Whall, A. (1996). The structure of nursing knowledge: Analysis and evaluation of practice, middle-range, and grand theory. In J. Fitzpatrick & A. Whall (Eds.), *Conceptual models of nursing: Analysis and application* (3rd ed., pp. 13–24). Stanford, CT: Appleton & Lange.

Wharton, E. (1904). The descent of man. From the *Oxford dictionary of 20th-century quotations* (p. 325). New York: Oxford University Press.

Wolanin, M., & Phillips, L. (1981). *Confusion: Prevention and care.* St. Louis: Mosby.

World Health Organization. (1974). *Chronicle of WHO, 1,* 1–2.

Yancey, P., & Brand, P. (1993). *The gift of pain.* Grand Rapids, MI: Zondervan Publishing (Previously titled *The Gift Nobody Wants.*)

Youngblut, J., & Casper, G. (1993). Single-item indicators in nursing research. *Research in Nursing and Health, 16,* 459–465.

Zerwekh, J. (1997). Do dying patients really need IV fluids? *American Journal of Nursing, 97*(3), 26–30.

General Comfort Questionnaire

Date _____   Code _____

Thank you VERY MUCH for helping us understand your COMFORT. Below are statements that relate to your comfort right now. Six numbers are provided for each question; please circle the number you think most closely matches your feeling. Your responses should describe your comfort *right now*.

		Strongly Disagree					Strongly Agree
1.	My body is relaxed right now	1	2	3	4	5	6
2.	I feel useful because I'm working hard	1	2	3	4	5	6
3.	I have enough privacy	1	2	3	4	5	6
4.	There are those I can depend on when I need help	1	2	3	4	5	6
5.	I don't want to exercise	1	2	3	4	5	6
6.	My condition gets me down	1	2	3	4	5	6
7.	I feel confident	1	2	3	4	5	6
8.	I feel dependent on others	1	2	3	4	5	6
9.	I feel my life is worthwhile right now	1	2	3	4	5	6

(continued)

		Strongly Disagree					Strongly Agree
10.	I am inspired by knowing that I am loved	1	2	3	4	5	6
11.	These surroundings are pleasant	1	2	3	4	5	6
12.	The sounds keep me from resting	1	2	3	4	5	6
13.	No one understands me	1	2	3	4	5	6
14.	My pain is difficult to endure	1	2	3	4	5	6
15.	I am inspired to do my best	1	2	3	4	5	6
16.	I am unhappy when I am alone	1	2	3	4	5	6
17.	My faith helps me to not be afraid	1	2	3	4	5	6
18.	I do not like it here	1	2	3	4	5	6
19.	I am constipated right now	1	2	3	4	5	6
20.	I do not feel healthy right now	1	2	3	4	5	6
21.	This room makes me feel scared	1	2	3	4	5	6
22.	I am afraid of what is next	1	2	3	4	5	6
23.	I am being treated fairly	1	2	3	4	5	6
24.	I have experienced changes which make me feel uneasy	1	2	3	4	5	6
25.	I am hungry	1	2	3	4	5	6
26.	I would like to see my doctor more often	1	2	3	4	5	6
27.	The temperature in this room is fine	1	2	3	4	5	6
28.	I am very tired	1	2	3	4	5	6
29.	I can rise above my pain	1	2	3	4	5	6
30.	The mood around here uplifts me	1	2	3	4	5	6
31.	I am content	1	2	3	4	5	6
32.	This chair (bed) makes me hurt	1	2	3	4	5	6
33.	My care is personalized	1	2	3	4	5	6
34.	My personal belongings are not here	1	2	3	4	5	6
35.	I feel out of place here	1	2	3	4	5	6
36.	I feel good enough to walk	1	2	3	4	5	6

		Strongly Disagree					Strongly Agree
37.	My friends/family remember me with their cards and phone calls	1	2	3	4	5	6
38.	My beliefs give me peace of mind	1	2	3	4	5	6
39.	I need to be better informed about my health	1	2	3	4	5	6
40.	I feel out of control	1	2	3	4	5	6
41.	I feel safe	1	2	3	4	5	6
42.	This room smells terrible	1	2	3	4	5	6
43.	I usually have to wait a long time for help	1	2	3	4	5	6
44.	I feel peaceful	1	2	3	4	5	6
45.	I am depressed	1	2	3	4	5	6
46.	I have found meaning in my life	1	2	3	4	5	6
47.	It is easy to get around here	1	2	3	4	5	6
48.	I need to feel good again	1	2	3	4	5	6

APPENDIX **B**

Radiation Therapy—Comfort Questionnaire

Date _____
Code _____

Thank you very much for helping me in my study of the concept comfort. Below are statements that may describe your comfort now. Six numbers are provided for each question; please circle the number you think most closely matches your feeling. Relate these questions to your comfort *at the moment you are answering the questions.*

		Strongly Agree					Strongly Disagree
1.	I feel lousy right now	6	5	4	3	2	1
2.	I feel good about myself	6	5	4	3	2	1
3.	It helps to talk to people about my cancer	6	5	4	3	2	1
4.	I am just as attractive physically as I always was	6	5	4	3	2	1

(continued)

		Strongly Agree					Strongly Disagree
5.	I feel fatigued	6	5	4	3	2	1
6.	I like the way the radiation department feels	6	5	4	3	2	1
7.	I don't have enough information about my cancer	6	5	4	3	2	1
8.	My breast feels normal	6	5	4	3	2	1
9.	I wonder if I made the right medical decision	6	5	4	3	2	1
10.	I have lost my appetite	6	5	4	3	2	1
11.	I do not worry about the equipment in the radiation department	6	5	4	3	2	1
12.	I don't like to be alone in the treatment room	6	5	4	3	2	1
13.	I am able to sleep well	6	5	4	3	2	1
14.	Life is worthwhile right now	6	5	4	3	2	1
15.	I am uneasy about the sounds that the radiation machines make	6	5	4	3	2	1
16.	There are those that I can depend on when I need help	6	5	4	3	2	1
17.	I have pain in my breast	6	5	4	3	2	1
18.	It is difficult to accept the idea that I had cancer	6	5	4	3	2	1
19.	I feel out of place in the radiation department	6	5	4	3	2	1
20.	No one understands me	6	5	4	3	2	1

		Strongly Agree					Strongly Disagree
21.	My skin around my breast and arm feels strong and healthy	6	5	4	3	2	1
22.	I feel out of control	6	5	4	3	2	1
23.	My friends remember me with their cards, phone calls, or letters	6	5	4	3	2	1
24.	I am afraid of what is next	6	5	4	3	2	1
25.	I think of the table I lie on for treatments as being hard and unfriendly	6	5	4	3	2	1
26.	I feel supported in my decision to have radiation therapy	6	5	4	3	2	1

Comfort Lines

Code # _____

Please place a dot on each of the four lines, corresponding to the level of agreement you feel right now with each statement next to the line.

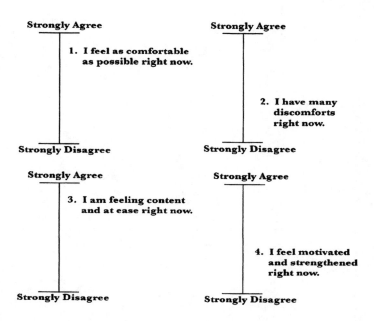

Strongly Agree

1. **I feel as comfortable as possible right now.**

Strongly Disagree

Strongly Agree

2. **I have many discomforts right now.**

Strongly Disagree

Strongly Agree

3. **I am feeling content and at ease right now.**

Strongly Disagree

Strongly Agree

4. **I feel motivated and strengthened right now.**

Strongly Disagree

Note: When reproducing these visual analogue scales, each should be 10 centimeters in length.

Peri-Operative Comfort Questionnaire

Code # _____

Thank you very much for your help with this comfort study. Below are statements that may describe your comfort associated with your surgery. Six numbers are provided for each question; please circle the number you think most closely matches your feeling.

		Strongly Disagree					Strongly Agree
1.	I was calm.	1	2	3	4	5	6
2.	I was cold.	1	2	3	4	5	6
3.	The environment was impersonal.	1	2	3	4	5	6
4.	My condition gets me down.	1	2	3	4	5	6
5.	My family/friends helped me to cope.	1	2	3	4	5	6
6.	I had a chance to speak with my anesthetist before surgery.	1	2	3	4	5	6

(continued)

		Strongly Disagree					Strongly Agree
7.	My modesty was not protected.	1	2	3	4	5	6
8.	My anxiety was high.	1	2	3	4	5	6
9.	The anesthesia personnel did not care about my feelings.	1	2	3	4	5	6
10.	The noises were disturbing.	1	2	3	4	5	6
11.	My anesthetist was gentle.	1	2	3	4	5	6
12.	I needed more information about my anesthesia.	1	2	3	4	5	6
13.	I felt out of control.	1	2	3	4	5	6
14.	The mood around here was reassuring.	1	2	3	4	5	6
15.	The quality of my care was poor.	1	2	3	4	5	6
16.	My wishes were carried out.	1	2	3	4	5	6
17.	My sense of self-respect was not preserved.	1	2	3	4	5	6
18.	I was able to visualize a successful recovery.	1	2	3	4	5	6
19.	The environment here felt safe.	1	2	3	4	5	6
20.	My care helped me feel confident.	1	2	3	4	5	6
21.	I was not afraid to go to sleep.	1	2	3	4	5	6
22.	My IV site was painful.	1	2	3	4	5	6
23.	I am satisfied with the care I received here.	1	2	3	4	5	6
24.	My anesthetist took good care of me.	1	2	3	4	5	6

Note to researcher: This can be converted to present tense if used to assess baseline comfort. Also, this instrument has not been tested.

Modified Karnofsky Performance Status Scale

100—no complaints, no evidence of disease

90—able to carry on normal work activity; minor signs and symptoms

80—normal activity with difficulty, in spite of signs and symptoms of disease

70—unable to carry on normal activity, in spite of signs and symptoms of disease

60—requires occasional assistance, but is able to be independent with ADLs; able to meet 60%–70% of own needs

50—requires considerable assistance and frequent medical care; needs assistance with ADLs

40—disabled; requires special care, maximum assistance, but can complete 20% of ADLs

30—severely disabled, although death is not imminent; unable to swallow

20—gravely ill; unable to swallow; totally dependent

10—actively dying

0—dead

Source: Karnofsky, D., & Burchenal, J. (1949). The clinical evaluation of chemotherapeutic agents against cancer. In N. McLeod (Ed.), *Evaluation of chemotherapeutic agents* (pp. 191–205). New York: Columbia University Press.

Hospice Comfort Questionnaire (Patient)

Date _____
Code # _____

Thank you very much for helping us in the study of hospice nursing. Below are statements that pertain to your comfort right now. Six numbers are provided for each question; please circle the number you think most closely matches your feeling. Relate these questions to your comfort *at the moment you are answering the questions.*

	Strongly Agree					Strongly Disagree
*1. **My body is relaxed right now**	6	5	4	3	2	1
*2. **My breathing is difficult**	6	5	4	3	2	1
3. I have enough privacy	6	5	4	3	2	1
*4. **There are those I can depend on when I need help**	6	5	4	3	2	1

(continued)

		Strongly Agree					Strongly Disagree
5.	I feel bloated	6	5	4	3	2	1
*6.	I worry about my family	6	5	4	3	2	1
7.	My beliefs give me peace of mind	6	5	4	3	2	1
8.	My nurse(s) give me hope	6	5	4	3	2	1
9.	My life is worthwhile right now	6	5	4	3	2	1
*10.	I know I am loved	6	5	4	3	2	1
*11.	These surroundings are pleasant	6	5	4	3	2	1
*12.	I have difficulty resting	6	5	4	3	2	1
13.	No one understands me	6	5	4	3	2	1
14.	My pain is difficult to endure	6	5	4	3	2	1
*15.	I feel peaceful	6	5	4	3	2	1
*16.	I sleep soundly	6	5	4	3	2	1
17.	I feel guilty	6	5	4	3	2	1
*18.	I like being here	6	5	4	3	2	1
*19.	I am nauseated	6	5	4	3	2	1
*20.	I am able to communicate with my loved ones	6	5	4	3	2	1
21.	This room makes me feel scared	6	5	4	3	2	1
*22.	I am afraid of what is next	6	5	4	3	2	1
23.	I have a special person(s) who make(s) me feel cared for	6	5	4	3	2	1
*24.	I have experienced changes that make me feel uneasy	6	5	4	3	2	1
25.	I like my room to be quiet	6	5	4	3	2	1
26.	I would like to see my doctor more often	6	5	4	3	2	1

	Strongly Agree					Strongly Disagree
*27. My mouth and skin feel very dry	6	5	4	3	2	1
*28. I am okay with my personal relationships	6	5	4	3	2	1
*29. I can rise above my pain	6	5	4	3	2	1
*30. The mood around here is depressing	6	5	4	3	2	1
31. I am at ease physically	6	5	4	3	2	1
*32. This chair/bed makes me hurt	6	5	4	3	2	1
33. This view inspires me	6	5	4	3	2	1
34. I think about my discomforts constantly	6	5	4	3	2	1
*35. I feel confident spiritually	6	5	4	3	2	1
*36. I feel good enough to do some things for myself	6	5	4	3	2	1
37. My friends remember me with their cards and phone calls	6	5	4	3	2	1
38. I feel out of place here	6	5	4	3	2	1
39. I need to be better informed about my condition	6	5	4	3	2	1
*40. I feel helpless	6	5	4	3	2	1
41. My God is helping me	6	5	4	3	2	1
42. This room smells fresh	6	5	4	3	2	1
*43. I feel lonely	6	5	4	3	2	1
44. I am able to tell people what I need	6	5	4	3	2	1
45. I am depressed	6	5	4	3	2	1

(continued)

	Strongly Agree					Strongly Disagree
46. I have found meaning in my life	6	5	4	3	2	1
*47. In retrospect, I've had a good life	6	5	4	3	2	1
48. My loved ones' state of mind makes me feel sad	6	5	4	3	2	1
49. The temperature in this room is fine	6	5	4	3	2	1

*Use only starred, bold items for a shorter questionnaire.

American Nurses Association Code of Ethics for Nurses

1. The nurse provides services with respect for human dignity and the uniqueness of the client, unrestricted by considerations of social or economic status, personal attributes, or the nature of health problems.
2. The nurse safeguards the client's right to privacy by judiciously protecting information of a confidential nature.
3. The nurse acts to safeguard the client and the public when health care and safety are affected by incompetent, unethical, or illegal practice by any person.
4. The nurse assumes accountability and responsibility for individual nursing judgments and actions.
5. The nurse maintains competence in nursing.
6. The nurse exercises informed judgment and uses individual competency and qualifications as criteria in seeking consultation, accepting responsibilities, and delegating nursing activities.
7. The nurse participates in activities that contribute to the ongoing development of the profession's body of knowledge.
8. The nurse participates in the profession's efforts to implement and improve standards of nursing.

(continued)

9. The nurse participates in the profession's efforts to establish and maintain conditions of employment conducive to high quality nursing care.
10. The nurse participates in the profession's efforts to protect the public from misinformation and misrepresentation and to maintain the integrity of nursing.
11. The nurse collaborates with members of the health care professions and other citizens in promoting community and national efforts to meet the health needs of the public.

Courtesy of the American Nurses Association (1985), Publication #G-56.

International Council of Nurses (ICN) Code of Ethics for Nurses

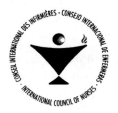

Preamble

Nurses have four fundamental responsibilities: to promote health, to prevent illness, to restore health and to alleviate suffering. The need for nursing is universal.

Inherent in nursing is respect for human rights, including the right to life, to dignity and to be treated with respect. Nursing care is unrestricted by considerations of age, colour, creed, culture, disability or illness, gender, nationality, politics, race or social status.

Nurses render health services to the individual, the family and the community and co-ordinate their services with those of related groups.

THE CODE

The ICN Code of Ethics for Nurses has four principal elements that outline the standards of ethical conduct.

Elements of the Code

1. Nurses and people

The nurse's primary professional responsibility is to people requiring nursing care.

In providing care, the nurse promotes an environment in which the human rights, values, customs and spiritual beliefs of the individual, family and community are respected.

The nurse ensures that the individual receives sufficient information on which to base consent for care and related treatment.

The nurse holds in confidence personal information and uses judgement in sharing this information.

The nurse shares with society the responsibility for initiating and supporting action to meet the health and social needs of the public, in particular those of vulnerable populations.

The nurse also shares responsibility to sustain and protect the natural environment from depletion, pollution, degradation and destruction.

2. Nurses and practice

The nurse carries personal responsibility and accountability for nursing practice, and for maintaining competence by continual learning.

The nurse maintains a standard of personal health such that the ability to provide care is not compromised.

The nurse uses judgement regarding individual competence when accepting and delegating responsibility.

The nurse at all times maintains standards of personal conduct which reflect well on the profession and enhance public confidence.

The nurse, in providing care, ensures that use of technology and scientific advances are compatible with the safety, dignity and rights of people.

3. Nurses and the profession

The nurse assumes the major role in determining and implementing acceptable standards of clinical nursing practice, management, research and education.

The nurse is active in developing a core of research-based professional knowledge.

The nurse, acting through the professional organisation, participates in creating and maintaining equitable social and economic working conditions in nursing.

4. Nurses and co-workers

The nurse sustains a co-operative relationship with co-workers in nursing and other fields.

The nurse takes appropriate action to safeguard individuals when their care is endangered by a co-worker or any other person.

FAQs From The Comfort Line

Below are frequently asked questions (FAQs) from my students and e-mail contacts. I have lifted this appendix from my Web site, *www. uakron.edu/comfort/*, after updating the FAQ section. Most of these questions are answered more fully in the text of the book, but may not be as easy to find. (If one wants to know how I arrived at my answers, the context can be found within the chapters.)

THEORETICAL DEVELOPMENT

1. *How do you define comfort for nursing research?*
   Holistic comfort is defined as the immediate experience of being strengthened through having the needs for Relief, Ease, and Transcendence met in four contexts of experience (physical, psychospiritual, sociocultural, and environmental). (Chapter 1)

2. *How do you define the types and contexts of comfort?*
   Types of Comfort: three components of comfort (factors or subscales)

   > *Relief:* the state of a patient who has had a specific need met.
   > *Ease:* the state of calm or contentment.
   > *Transcendence:* the state in which one rises above one's problems or pain.

Contexts in Which Comfort Is Experienced: how comfort is experienced or perceived; causes of or detractors from comfort

Physical: pertaining to bodily sensations and homeostatic mechanisms.

Psychospiritual: pertaining to internal awareness of self, including esteem, concept, sexuality, and meaning in one's life; one's relationship to a higher order or being.

Environmental: pertaining to external surroundings, conditions, and influences.

Sociocultural: pertaining to interpersonal, family, and societal relationships. Also to family traditions, rituals, and religious practices.

3. *Why do you combine psychological comfort and spiritual comfort into one context of experience called "psychospiritual"?*
   They were combined because indicators of each overlapped and, in some cases, were identical (e.g., meaningfulness, faith, identity, self-esteem). Judith Spross independently combined psychological and spiritual contexts the same way and came up with the same contexts of experience in her work about suffering. (Chapter 1)

4. *What is the relationship between comfort and pain?*
   Comfort is a larger umbrella term compared to pain. As stated above, there are three types of comfort: Relief, Ease, and Transcendence. Relief is the absence of specific previous discomforts, a common one being pain which can be of varying intensity. Pain that has a physical origin is also influenced by psychospiritual, sociocultural, and environmental factors.

   I define pain as a multidimensional discomfort including sensory, cognitive, and affective components (Melzak & Wall, 1982). It is a specific sensation in the body that "hurts" with a varying degree of intensity (for example, from mild to severe or from 1 to 10). The discomfort of pain is often a significant detractor from comfort. (The concepts of comfort, discomfort, and pain are defined in Glossary.)

5. *What nurse theorists are incorporated into your conceptualization of comfort?*
   Relief: Orlando (1961/1990)
   Ease: Henderson (1978)
   Transcendence: Paterson and Zderad (1976/1988)

Contexts of comfort come from nursing literature on holism. (Chapter 1)

6. *Why is your definition of comfort so complicated?*
   Comfort is a complex concept but, prior to this work, was defined negatively as an absence of discomforts such as pain, nausea, and itching (Funk, Tornquist, Champagne, Copp, & Wies, 1989). My definition characterizes comfort as a positive concept and accounts for its many aspects beyond physical comfort. The taxonomic structure enables us to identify comfort needs, design interventions (comfort measures) targeted to those needs, and measure the effectiveness of those interventions. (Chapter 1)

7. *How did you get started in your study of comfort?*
   An early assignment in my MSN program (by Dr. Rosemary Ellis) was to diagram my nursing practice. At that time, I was a head nurse on an Alzheimer's unit and I used the concept of comfort to designate the state I wanted my patients to have when they weren't trying to perform special tasks. At a presentation of my "framework" to a gerontological conference, I was asked if I had done a concept analysis of comfort. I replied, "No, but that's the next step." Actually, I hadn't thought about it before, but realized that it should be my next step (this demonstrates the value of presenting your ideas and being open to feedback). Thereafter, I felt that I had an obligation to do the concept analysis after committing myself publicly. (That was 15 years ago!) (Chapter 1)

8. *Why do you call your theory a "mid-range" Theory of Comfort?*
   This is not a broad or grand theory. The working part of the theory is found on the *last* full line of each conceptual framework (Figures 5.2 and 9.1) which shows the relationships between measurable and defined concepts. Also, the theory can be easily operationalized for appropriate settings. When each concept is operationalized, you have a practice level theory. (Chapters 5, 7, and 9)

9. *How do you define the metaparadigm concepts?*
   Nursing: the intentional assessment of comfort needs, design of comfort measures to address those needs, and reassessment of patients' or community's comfort after implementation of

comfort measures, compared to a previous baseline.
Patient: an individual, family, community, or country in need of health care.
Environment: an aspect of patient/family comfort that can be manipulated to enhance comfort.
Health: optimum function of a patient/family/community/country facilitated by enhanced comfort. (Chapter 4)

10. *What is borrowed and what is unique about Comfort Theory?*
    I borrowed the ideas about Relief, Ease, and Transcendence as stated in the answer to question 5. Later, I borrowed the contexts of experience from the literature review about holism. I put these ideas together in a unique way. Later still, I borrowed the framework for the first and second parts of Comfort Theory from Henry Murray (see comfort theory article). But I hung nursing concepts on his abstract framework in a unique way. The idea of Institutional Integrity was unique (I made it up!) and it was added through a process Tomey and Alligood call retroduction. (Chapters 4 and 9)

11. *Can Comfort Theory be used in different cultures?*
    Patient comfort has been described in Canadian, Hispanic, and Australian cultures. In addition, I have had inquiries from Iran, Turkey, Thailand, China, South America, Norway, and other countries. I have concluded that comfort is a universal concept. The first step to testing comfort theory in other cultures is to translate the instrument into a different language. I am looking for volunteers! (Chapter 10)

12. *On a continuum, what is the opposite of comfort?*
    I believe the opposite of comfort is suffering. (Chapter 6)

13. *What are the latest developments with Comfort Theory?*
    I added the concept and definition of institutional outcomes to the theory to address the trend in nursing research and practice to measure outcomes of nursing care. I also changed social comfort to sociocultural comfort. (Chapter 9)

EDUCATION AND PRACTICE

1. *Isn't Comfort Care impractical in a downsized setting?*
   Comfort Care is efficient and satisfying to patients and nurses;

thus, it is even more important in a time of limited resources. Plus, Comfort Care offers a framework for making nurses recognizable and indispensable because of what they do. When patients and families associate enhanced comfort with Registered Nurses, they will *demand* that RNs are readily available. (Chapter 9)

Also, Comfort Care is a framework for interdisciplinary health care, as it focuses on patients. As such it is a unifying framework for care for the future.

Note: When presenting comfort care to students a few years ago, one earnest young man who had some prior experience working in nursing homes raised his hand and asked, "Is this a new concept? I have never seen it being practiced!" I think his question is a wake-up call to us in nursing practice and education to get back to the basics.

2. *Is Comfort Care difficult to learn?*
No. Comfort Care is intuitive because we are all familiar with our own comfort. The template for Comfort Care can be applied repeatedly but individualistically to most patients, so that it becomes automatic, thorough, and satisfying. (Chapters 9 and 10)

3. *Does the framework of Comfort Care account for medical problems and/ or pain that patients experience?*
Yes. Physical comfort includes balance in oxygenation, elimination, mobility, cognitive abilities, electrolyte balance, pain management, hydration, and all aspects of the medical problem(s). (Chapter 5)

4. *Care plans are becoming obsolete. Are there other teaching/learning (heuristic) devices for students?*
Yes. On clinical preparation sheets, students can identify comfort needs in four contexts: physical (see question 3 above), psychospiritual, sociocultural, and environmental. Students should list, in another section, the intervening variables so that a full picture of each patient emerges. Then, they can list interventions, patients' perception of comfort after the interventions, what the nurse does next, realistic health seeking behaviors, and expected institutional outcomes (patient satisfaction is the easiest). (Chapters 9 and 10)

RESEARCH

1. *What was the topic of your dissertation?*
    I did a pilot study of the General Comfort Questionnaire while in graduate school. At CWRU, I was told, this was not sufficient for graduation. My advisor then "suggested" I do an intervention study to see if comfort was really measurable. Therefore, I chose a population of people who had acute comfort needs (women with early-stage breast cancer), a holistic intervention that was practical for implementation (audiotaped guided imagery), and three repeated measures in order to demonstrate a trend if any existed. I graduated in December, 1996 after 11 years in the doctoral program at FPB. (Eleven years sounds awful but I took one course at a time while working full time at The University of Akron and raising a family.) My dissertation is available from CWRU (Kolcaba, 1998) and in an article published in *Oncology Nursing Forum* (Kolcaba & Fox, 1999).

2. *What statistical method do you recommend for comfort research?*
    Because comfort theoretically is state-specific, it should be measured prior to one's intervention and at least two times after the intervention. Repeated Measures MANCOVA is recommended for statistical analysis because time is used as a contrast on the mean of the dependent variables (your measurements of comfort at each time point). Also, subjects serve as their own controls. Trend analysis can be used to demonstrate the model of differences in comfort over time between treatment and control groups.
    Data from visual analog scales can be computed the same way. Our visual analog scales (Comfort Lines) are 10 centimeters/ 100 millimeters long and we use four of them to measure Total Comfort, Relief, Ease, and Transcendence. After reverse coding Relief, measure from the bottom the number of millimeters for each scale (e.g., 6.40 cmms. or 64 mms.). To obtain reliability figures, do test-retest procedures about 10 minutes apart. (Test-retest reliability is not appropriate when considerable time has elapsed, especially in stressful health care situations, because the state of comfort is too variable.)

3. *What research are you currently working on?*
    My research partner, Dr. Therese Dowd, has been interested in

urinary incontinence (UI) and urinary frequency (UF) for a long time (we call it compromised urinary bladder syndrome or CUBS). She asked me if my theory was compatible with that condition. Since I think that adult or childhood UI and UF detracts from holistic comfort, I said "Definitely!" Therefore, we are immersed in a research program to target the multiple health care needs of persons with UI/UF. We design interventions to meet those needs, such as bladder health information and cognitive strategies, and measure comfort (Urinary Incontinence and Frequency Comfort Questionnaire [Dowd, Kolcaba, & Steiner, 2000]) as the immediate desired outcome with several other health seeking behaviors as the subsequent outcomes (perception of health, quality of life, and episodes of UI/UF). Currently, we are applying our findings to persons in assisted living situations and eventually, in long-term care settings.

Another program of research is end-of-life comfort. A study we are just beginning is the efficacy of hand/wrist massage on comfort and associated outcomes for persons near end of life. We will use the End of Life Comfort Questionnaire (Novak, Kolcaba, Steiner, & Dowd, 2001). This is a difficult research setting, but we have worked with this population before and are fairly aware of the issues that arise and are working hard to compensate for them. (Chapter 9)

A third topic of interest, which I am just beginning to explore, is outcomes associated with Parish Nursing.

All of our work will be available from Springer Publishing or from my Web site.

4. *Can I ask you questions about developing my research design?*
   Yes. Just use my e-mail address [kolcaba@uakron.edu.] which I check frequently. I always appreciate your interest, questions, and feedback even if you decide not to use Comfort Theory.

Evaluation of Comfort Theory

The following criteria for evaluation of a nursing theory came from the 5th edition of *Nursing Theorists and Their Work* by Tomey and Alligood (2001). These responses to the criteria were written by Dr. Therese Dowd, my research partner and are used with permission of the publisher, Mosby (2001, pp. 439–440).

CLARITY

Some of the early articles, such as the concept analysis piece, are difficult to read but are consistent in terms of definitions, derivations, assumptions, and propositions. The seminal article explicating the Theory of Comfort is easier to read and, in subsequent articles, Kolcaba applies the theory to specific practices utilizing academic but understandable and consistent language. All concepts are theoretically and operationally defined.

SIMPLICITY

The Theory of Comfort is simple in so far as it harkens to basic nursing care and the traditional mission of nursing. It is low-tech in language and application, but this does not preclude its usage in high-tech settings. There are few variables in the theory and not all the variables have to be utilized for any research or educational project. The main thrust of the theory is to return nursing to a practice focused on needs of patients, inside or outside institutional walls. Because of its simplicity and intuitive appeal, the theory is easily learned and practiced by students and practicing nurses.

GENERALITY

Kolcaba's theory has been applied in numerous research settings, cultures, and age groups. The only limiting factor for its application is how much commitment nurses and administrations are willing to make for meeting the comfort needs of patients. If both the nurse and the institution/community are committed to this type of health care, the Theory of Comfort enables nurses and the health care team to practice in efficient, individualized, holistic patterns. The TS of comfort allows researchers to develop their own comfort interventions and instruments for new settings.

EMPIRICAL PRECISION

The first part of the theory, predicting that effective nursing interventions offered over time will demonstrate enhanced comfort, has been tested and supported with women with breast cancer (Kolcaba & Fox, 1999) and persons with urinary incontinence (UI) (Dowd, Kolcaba, & Steiner, 2000). In the UI study, enhanced comfort also was related to an increase in HSBs, supporting the second part of the comfort theory. The relationship between comfort and institutional integrity currently is being tested.

For patients with breast cancer and UI, plus for those at end of life (Novak, Kolcaba, Dowd, & Steiner, 2001) the adapted comfort instruments have shown strong psychometric properties, meaning that those questionnaires are reliable and valid measurements of comfort and can demonstrate changes in comfort over time. These findings support the theoretical foundation for the taxonomic structure of comfort.

DERIVABLE CONSEQUENCES

The Theory of Comfort describes a patient-centered practice. It is important to determine if comfort measures matter to patients, their health, and the viability of institutions. The theory also predicts the benefits of effective interventions for enhancing comfort and facilitating engagement in HSBs. The Theory of Comfort is dedicated to strengthening nursing while bringing the discipline back in contact with its roots. But it can be utilized by other health care professionals such as physicians, social workers, psychologists, clergy, nursing assistants, and auxiliary personnel.

In addition, specific criteria for evaluating *mid-range* theories were applied to Comfort Theory. They are: (1) its concepts and propositions are specific to nursing, (2) it is readily operationalized, (3) it can be applied to many situations, (4) propositions can range from causal to associative, depending on their application, and (5) assumptions fit the theory. These are characteristics of good MR theory as described by Whall (1996). Nolan and Grant (1992) suggested two additional criteria if a theory is to be practical in practice. Those criteria are (6) it should be relevant for potential users of the theory, i.e., nurses, and (7) it should be oriented to outcomes that are important for patients, not merely describe what nurses do. The Mid-Range Theory of Comfort fulfills these seven criteria.

Glossary

Alpha Press—the sum of negative (obstructing) forces, positive (facilitating) forces, and interacting forces (*see* Murray's Theory of Human Press)

Assumptions—an author's understanding about reality

Autonomy—acting or making choices for oneself

Beneficence—an ethic of "doing nice things" because they ought to be done

Best Interest Principle—the ethical rule stating that when an incapacitated patient has not discussed his/her treatment preferences with the surrogate, the surrogate must apply general knowledge of the patient and the patient's values to treatment decisions (Robinson, 2001)

Beta Press—the patient's perception of how well health care interventions (facilitating forces) met the needs arising from the health care situation (obstructing forces) for which the patient required assistance to satisfy; the person's *perception* of the total effect of the forces in alpha press (*see* Murray's Theory of Human Press)

CINAHL (Cumulative Index of Nursing and Allied Health Literature)—a large research data base for health researchers available through university libraries on the Web

Clinical Ladders—a process available to nurses in some institutions where a small study or project, successfully completed, is part of a system of career progression

Coaching—*see* Comfort Measures

Comfort—the immediate experience of being strengthened by having needs for relief, ease, and transcendence met in four contexts (physical, psychospiritual, social, and environmental); much more than the absence of pain (Kolcaba)

Comfort Care—a philosophy of health care that focuses on addressing physical (including homeostatic mechanisms as well as sensations), psychospiritual, sociocultural, and environmental comfort needs of patients. Comfort Care has three components: (a) an appropriate and timely intervention, (b) a mode of delivery that projects caring and empathy, and (c) the intent to comfort (Kolcaba, 1995a)

Comfort Diner—a vision for a national human environment that intentionally values and facilitates comfort and health of its citizens through equity of access, cost, professionalism, caring, technology, support, respect, and dignity (Kolcaba)

Comfort Food for the Soul—*see* Comfort Measures

Comfort Grid—*see* Taxonomic Structure

Comfort Measures—interventions designed intentionally to enhance patients' comfort
    technical comfort measures—interventions designed to maintain homeostasis and manage pain, such as monitoring blood chemistries, vital signs, and administering pain medications
    coaching—interventions designed to relieve anxiety, provide reassurance and information, instill hope, listen, and help plan realistically for recovery, integration, or death in a culturally sensitive way; consist usually of active listening, touch, and positive reinforcement
    comfort food for the soul—interventions that are not expected, are not technical, and are, perhaps, "old-fashioned" that make patients feel strengthened in an intangible, personalized sort of way (e.g., back massage)

Comfort Line—Kolcaba's Web site at *www.uakron.edu/comfort*

Comfort Needs—a desire for or deficit in relief/ease/transcendence in physical, psychospiritual, sociocultural, and environmental contexts of human experience

Concept Analysis—examining the parts of a term or word to determine how they are interrelated and organized; includes a precise definition of that term

Conceptual Definition—statement about the meaning of a word in plain language; can be a technical definition (more precise and complicated, often specific to a profession)

Concurrent Validity—the extent to which a measure correlates with another simultaneously obtained measure of the same trait or state (Goodwin & Goodwin, 1991)

Construct—an umbrella for several concepts; comfort could be called a construct because it contains the concepts of relief, ease, and transcendence (For simplicity, however, I use the term concept.)

Contexts of Comfort—how comfort is experienced or perceived; causes of comfort
    Physical Comfort—pertaining to bodily sensations and homeostatic mechanisms that may or may not be related to specific diagnoses
    Psychospiritual Comfort—whatever gave life meaning for an individual and entailed self-esteem, self-concept, sexuality, and his/her relationship to a higher order or being
    Environmental Comfort—pertaining to external surroundings, conditions, and influences
    Sociocultural Comfort—pertaining to interpersonal, family, and societal relationships including finances, education, and support, including family histories, traditions, language, clothes, and customs

Data Sets—integrated, computerized, clinical informational systems used for outcomes research about interventions and outcomes, usually specific to a particular practice within health care
    Nursing Outcomes Classification (NOC)—a systematic listing of outcomes that measure the effectiveness of nursing interventions
    Nursing Intervention Classification (NIC)—a systematic listing of common nursing interventions

Deduction—form of logical reasoning in which specific conclusions are inferred from more general premises or principles; proceeds from the general to the specific (Bishop, 1998)

Discomfort—a physical, psychospiritual, sociocultural, or environmental detractor from comfort

Ease—a state of calm or contentment

Ecology—a hierarchy of domains in which living organisms respond and interact (species, communities, ecosystems, biospheres)

Entrusted Care—health care in which major and minor decisions for treatment are made by a surrogate

Environment—aspects of patient/family/community surroundings that affect comfort and can be manipulated to enhance comfort

Environmental Comfort—*see* Contexts of Comfort

Ethics—the study of conduct and chosen behavior
    ethics of obligation—when persons employ principles of conduct in making decisions; common morality; the difference between right and wrong; has intellectual and emotional components; includes rules or codes
    consequentialist ethics—when persons utilize estimates of the consequences of proposed actions to weigh alternatives; the action that promises the best consequences (outcomes) and is judged to be right
    ethics of virtue—when persons utilize their own character traits to assist with reasoning and motivating action

Excess Disabilities (EDs)—reversible symptoms in true dementia that are undesirable and temporary extensions of a specific primary disability (Schwab, Rader, & Doan, 1985)
    Physical—agitation, fear, or acting out caused by an infection, pain or discomfort, loss of homeostatsis, or other medical problems
    Psychological—agitation, fear, or acting out caused by mental or emotional discomforts

Facilitative Environment—the therapeutic milieu that is adapted to address the needs of frail patients (Wolanin & Phillips, 1981)

Facilitating Forces—nursing interventions designed to meet the needs that remain after the person's own reserves are depleted by obstructing forces (*see* Murray's Theory of Human Press)

Failure to Rescue—the death among patients caused by sepsis, pneumonia, shock, upper gastrointestinal bleeding, deep vein thrombosis (DVT), or other complications of hospitalization (HRSA, 2001)

Good Death—*see* peaceful death

Grand Theories—conceptual frameworks at a high level of abstraction, with many concepts that are not immediately measurable

Healing—what the patient or loved one needs to do at any given time, including feeling empowered to die peacefully or let a loved one go (Kolcaba); the emergence of right relationship at, between, and among all levels of human being (Watson, 1992, p. 28)

Healing Environment—an environment that facilitates "the emergence of the Haelan effect, the synergistic, organismic multidimensional response of whole persons in the direction of healing and wholeness" (Watson, 1992, p. 28)

Health—optimum function of a patient/family/community/country facilitated by enhanced comfort (Kolcaba, K., 1997)

Health Seeking Behaviors (HSBs)—behaviors in which patients engage consciously or subconsciously which move them toward well-being; HSBs can be internal, external, or a peaceful death (Schlotfeldt, 1975)

Holism—the belief that whole persons consist of a mental/spiritual/emotional life that is intimately connected with their physical bodies; persons' bodies comprise their own natural boundaries (Kolcaba, R., 1997)

Hope—the belief in a personal and better tomorrow and the expectation that a better tomorrow is truly possible and important

Human Press—*see* Murray's Theory of Human Press

Induction—process of building generalizations from a number of specific observed instances (Bishop, 1998)

Institutional Integrity (InI)—the quality or state of health care organizations being complete, whole, sound, upright, professional, and ethical providers of health care (Dowd, 2001; Kolcaba, 2001)

Intervening Variables—factors over which nurses or agencies have little control, but which affect the direction and success of Comfort Care plans or comfort studies

Magnet Organizations—health care institutions and agencies that demonstrate best practices in creating positive working environments for nurses and other members of the health care team (American Nurses Association, 2001)

Memorable Nurses—especially virtuous nurses whose ministration of comfort measures are above and beyond the call of duty and who are held in high esteem and gratefulness by patients and/or family members after the health care episode is completed

Metaparadigm—in nursing, the concepts central to the discipline (Fawcett, 1984); the concepts that Fawcett explicated are person, health, environment, and nursing

Mid-Range (MR) Theories—conceptual frameworks at a low level of abstraction that contain a small number of measurable concepts and relationships; they are adaptable to a wide range of practice and experience, can be built from many sources, and are concrete enough to be tested (Whall, 1996)

Murray's (1938) Theory of Human Press—general theory about human personality and needs that served as a framework from which Kolcaba's Mid-Range Theory of Comfort was substructed

Mythic Vision—an ideal of how human communities can live; a mythic vision evokes energies needed to sustain human effort involved in working toward common goals and values; it is highly romanticized if taken too literally, but is necessary for providing a context of a better world (Berry, 1988)

Needs—drives induced by obstructing forces that promote activities designed to satisfy the drives (Murray, 1938)

Nursing—the intentional assessment of comfort needs, design of comfort measures (interventions) to address those needs, and reassessment of patients' or community comfort after implementation of comfort measures, compared to a previous baseline (Kolcaba, K., 1997)

Nursing Sensitive Outcomes—results of health care that can be directly related to the interventions of professional nurses

Objective Data—observations made by the health care team to determine patient status

Obstructing Forces—the total negative stimuli arising from health care situations including side effects of illness or treatments, noxious or threatening environmental and social experiences, and emotional sensations such as fear, anxiety, powerlessness, or aloneness (*see* Murray's Theory of Human Press)

Operational Definition—a way in which a researcher measures a concept, usually in the form of a questionnaire, interview, or scale

Optimum Function—the ability to engage in special or challenging activities (Wolanin & Phillips, 1981)

Outcomes—results of health care interventions
　　diagnosis specific outcomes—results of patient care that are attributed to diagnosis, age, functional status upon admission, etc. (Johnson & Maas, 1999)

discipline specific outcomes—results of patient care that are attributed to specific health care professions, such as medical care (Johnson & Maas, 1999)

global outcomes—broad results of patient care that cannot be attributed to any one discipline, such as health status or patient satisfaction (Johnson & Maas, 1999)

negative outcomes—results of patient care that are undesirable, such as nosocomial infection

nursing sensitive outcomes—results of patient care that can be attributed to good nursing care, such as comfort (one type of discipline specific outcome)

positive outcomes—results of patient care that are desirable, such as early discharge

outcomes research—statistical analyses of large data sets that reveal the numbers of positive and negative outcomes attributable to specific institutions or disciplines

system specific outcomes—results of patient care that reflect organizational factors or geographic settings (Johnson & Maas, 1999)

Outcomes Research—analyses of large databases in an institution or geographically bounded area, about patterns and results of health care delivery

Pain—a multidimensional discomfort including sensory, cognitive, and affective components (Melzak & Wall, 1982); specific sensation in the body that hurts with a varying degree of intensity (for example, from mild to severe or from 1 to 10); the discomfort of pain is often a significant detractor from comfort

focal pain—a specific, severe, expected, and relatively localized pain associated with a surgical procedure, other pathology, or labor and delivery

pain intensifiers—responses that heighten the perception of pain within the conscious mind (Yancey & Brand, 1997)

Paradigm—world view, general philosophical perspective about reality

Patient—an individual, family, or community in need of health care (Kolcaba, K., 1997)

Peaceful Death—a death in which conflicts are resolved, symptoms are well managed, and acceptance by the patient and family members allows for the patient to "let go" quietly and with dignity

Physical Comfort—*see* Contexts of Comfort

Post-Hoc Tests—secondary statistical tests done after the primary statistical test, and only if the primary test is significant

Process—a method of doing something, with all steps involved; specifies a product or outcome (Webster, 1995)

Product—the result of the process, or that which is produced (Webster, 1995)

Productivity (nursing)—the extent to which a nurse or set of nurses achieve positive patient outcomes such as comfort, quick healing, early ambulation, return to previous function, adherence to a rehabilitation plan (*without* a quick readmission for the same medical problem), and patient satisfaction

Psychometric Properties—reliability and validity of instruments used for research, established through pilot testing and repeated use

Psychospiritual Comfort—*see* Contexts of Comfort

Quality of Life—a commonly used outcome of patient care that designates contentment about one's place in society and ability to function within desired roles; extent of feelings about one's well-being

Relief—the experience of a patient who has had a specific comfort need met

Renewal—*see* Transcendence

Repeated Measures Multivariate Analyses of Covariance (RM MAN-COVA)—the test statistic that looks at group differences, over time, and the interaction effects between time and group; baseline data serves as each subjects' own control

Retroduction—a form of reasoning that originates ideas

Sociocultural Comfort—*see* Contexts of Comfort

Stimulus Situation—alpha press and beta press arising from any health care situation (*see* Murray's Theory of Human Press)

Subjective Data—statements, body language, and behaviors of a patient that reveal his or her health status

Substituted Judgment—the ethical principle stating that in the absence of a written directive, a surrogate can come to the same decision the patient would if (s)he were not incapacitated (Robinson, 2001)

Successful Discharge—patients who avoid readmission to the hospital within 6 months for problems related to the condition(s) causing the original hospitalization

Supererogation—actions that go above and beyond what duty prescribes in a given profession

Supporting Data—facts from a patient's chart such as lab values, progress notes, vital signs, or reports that give clues to his/her health status

Technical Comfort Measures—*see* Comfort Measures

Taxonomic Structure (TS)—a 12-cell grid that depicts the content domain of comfort. The 12 cells result when the types of comfort (Relief, Ease, and Transcendence [across the top]) are juxtaposed with contexts of comfort (Physical, Psychospiritual, Sociocultural, and Environmental). The TS is used to identify comfort needs of a given population of patients, design interventions to meet those needs, and design Comfort Questionnaires (congruent with the intervention(s)) to measure change in comfort over time; contains the attributes of comfort

Technical Definition—statement about the meaning of a word in plain language, but is usually rather precise and specific to a profession

Thema—patterns of successful habits and goals that provide persons with direction for future action (*see* Murray's Theory of Human Press)

Theoretical Definition—*see* Conceptual Definition

Transcendence—the state in which one rises above problems or pain

Trend Analysis—a post hoc statistical test that tells one whether group differences follow a pattern; the pattern we found in our comfort studies was that the differences between groups were nonsignificant at Time 1, but that differences then got larger at Time 2 and still larger at Time 3. When the groups were plotted on two lines, the comparison group remained relatively flat while the line for the treatment group went up.

T-test—a statistical test that determines differences between groups on selected outcomes, such as comfort

Type I error—the possibility of finding significance when significance would be incorrect

Type II error—the possibility of failing to find significance when failing to do so would be incorrect

Types of Comfort—three components of comfort (factors or subscales), Relief, Ease, and Transcendence, that may or may not be present simultaneously

Unitary Trend—self-evaluations of outcomes in given situations that accumulate and provide the expectation that other situations will end similarly (*see* Murray's Theory of Human Press)

Visual Analog Scale—a type of questionnaire that consists of a line, usually 10 centimeters long, with anchors at either end such as "strongly agree" at one end and "strongly disagree" on the other end (example in Appendix C). The line can be vertical or horizontal, but we found patients near end of life did better with vertical lines, as they were similar to a thermometer concept (with higher comfort at top)

Well-being—extent and perception of quality of life

Index